The
Juicing
Book

Stephen Blauer

Foreword by Dr. Bernard Jensen

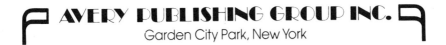

AVERY PUBLISHING GROUP INC.
Garden City Park, New York

The medical and health procedures in this book are based on the training, personal experiences, and research of the author. Because each person and situation is unique, the publisher urges the reader to check with a qualified health professional before using any procedure where there is any question as to its appropriateness.

The publisher does not advocate the use of any particular diet and exercise program, but believes the information presented in this book should be available to the public.

Because there is always some risk involved, the author and publisher are not responsible for any adverse effects or consequences resulting from the use of any of the suggestions, preparations, or procedures in this book. Please do not use the book if you are unwilling to assume the risk. Feel free to consult a physician or other qualified health professional. It is a sign of wisdom, not cowardice, to seek a second or third opinion.

Cover Designers: Rudy Shur and Martin Hochberg
Cover Photographer: Murray Alcosser
Illustrator: Vicky Hudon
In-House Editor: Nancy Marks Papritz

Library of Congress Cataloging-in-Publication Data

Blauer, Stephen.
    The juicing book / Stephen Blauer
        p.   cm.
    Includes index.
    ISBN 0-89529-253-X : $8.95
    1. Fruit juices--Therapeutic use.   2. Vegetable juices-
-Therapeutic use.   I. Title.
RM237.B57   1989   89-6725
613.2'6--dc20   CIP

Printed in the United States of America

10   9   8   7   6   5   4

Contents

Preface

The Elements of a
Long and Healthy Life

Fresh-juices are fantastic! As Nature's own nutrient-packed thirst quenchers, cleansers, and tonics, they can't be beat. Yet, as good as fresh-squeezed juices are, they are but one aspect of a healthy lifestyle. The greatest benefits of fresh juices are derived by combining them with a wholesome diet and a regular exercise program.

Most of us are born with the potential to live long, healthy, and happy lives. Why then do some of us fall short? There are at least three reasons.

The first reason is our belief system. We believe that as we age we become helpless and sickly—even though we see examples of youthful and energetic seniors all around us. It is important to believe in the examples of people whose health and longevity at advanced age seems remarkable. Their vitality is not an anomaly. It is our birthright.

The second reason we fall short of our potential is our lack of consistency. By not adhering to a lifelong regimen of wholesome diet and regular exercise, we do little to foster our own health and longevity. It is not what we eat or drink occasionally, but rather what we consume on a daily basis, that determines our level of health. That's why it is important to choose the freshest, most wholesome foods; those that are locally grown are best. It is equally important to find fresh, clean, spring water with which to drink and cook. And we must try to be active each day.

Our bodies thrive on moderate exercise, sunshine, and fresh air. That's why we should try to go outdoors daily and, whenever possible, go to places where we can marvel at the wonders of Nature. We can walk, run, play tennis or basketball, swim, mountain climb, or ski. Or we can try gardening, chopping wood, building, or other active and enjoyable hobbies.

The third reason we may fall short of our potential is that many of us hold an unfocused picture of the quality of our lives. For as the quality of life becomes unfocused, often so does life itself. Therefore, being conscious of the quality of our life is essential if we wish it to improve. A life filled with quality in work, thoughts, companions, and activities can strengthen our natural immunity to germs, viruses, and negative hereditary influences.

Lessons on longevity and happiness can be found by studying the lives of modern-day peoples who live in traditional cultures. Perhaps the most prolific examples of long life are found among the Hunzakut of Pakistan, the Vilcabamban of Ecuador, and the Abhasian of the Soviet Union. As individual groups, these societies enjoy a greater degree of immunity from illnesses of almost every type. They live closer to Nature in the foods they eat, in their work, and in their play habits. Conversely, Western society has strayed from Nature and somewhat from the intuitive ability to choose the foods, work, and habits that will bring its members true health, happiness, and long life.

The return to wholesome foods and fresh juices can be your first step on the journey to a more healthy and happy life. I hope this book will help you to take that first step.

Foreword
Variety is Key

I am delighted with the publication of *The Juicing Book*.

During my more than fifty-eight years in the healing art as a clinical nutritionist, I have seen hundreds of dietary fads come and go. Juices were not among them. Why? Because juices are not a fad. Juices are here to stay.

The fresh juices of fruits and vegetables are a food—an important, nutrient-rich, health-enhancing food. I've recommended fresh juice to my patients from my earliest days, and I still recommend juices, for very good reasons.

In my professional experience, I consider nutritional deficiencies to be among the most common and least acknowledged contributors to the development of disease and illness in our time, because so many people are not using balanced food programs centered around whole, pure, and natural foods, as they should.

Fresh fruit and vegetable juices contain a broad array of vitamins, minerals, enzymes, and various co-factors that both enhance and complement individual nutrients, so your body gets the most good from them. Because juices are assimilated with very little effort on the part of the digestive system, their nutrients have a health-building impact at a relatively low cost in energy. What this means is that juices are excellent for you whether your health and energy are at a low ebb right now or whether you've never felt better in your life.

This is not to say that adding more fresh juices to your diet will compensate for poor day-to-day nutrition habits. Rather, by adding fresh juices to a balanced food regimen, you will help accelerate and enhance the process of restoring nutrients to chemically-starved tissues. It is on these very tissues that disease and illness thrive. In terms of prevention, therefore, the importance of juice cannot be overstressed.

I believe in fresh juices. I have always considered fresh juices to be a necessary part of my Health and Harmony Food Regimen, a nutrition program that has helped thousands of my patients get well and stay well.

Perhaps because I live in the heart of California's citrus belt, people expect me to recommend orange juice over everything else. Let me share an important secret with you.

Variety is one of the most important, yet least practiced, food laws of Nature. *We need to eat a variety of proteins, starches, fruits, vegetables, and juices to prevent disease and build health.* Our bodies need a broad array of nutrients to defend against disease and to sustain well-being. *We need a variety of juices!*

My advice to you is this: enjoy reading this book, make practical use of this book, and use the many different varieties of fresh juices featured in this book to supplement and enhance your diet. You'll be glad you did.

Dr. Bernard Jensen
Escondido, California

Introduction
Juice Fact and Fiction

Americans are well acquainted with juices. We begin our days with orange juice, or grapefruit juice, or maybe a taste of prune juice. Both canned and bottled juices are popular at snack time and meal time. Quality-conscious consumers have created a market for commercially produced, 100-percent-natural juices. To round out their juice lines, manufacturers now offer several all-natural fruit juice blends from concentrate.

With all this attention focused on juices, why write a book on them? And, for that matter, why read one? Because drinking fresh juices is an excellent health habit that cannot be reinforced enough. Fresh juice is more than an excellent source of vitamins, minerals, enzymes, purified water, proteins, carbohydrates, and chlorophyll. Because it is in liquid form, fresh juice supplies nutrition that is not wasted to fuel its own digestion as it is with whole fruits, vegetables, and grasses. As a result, the body can quickly and easily make maximum use of all the nutrition that fresh juice offers.

Most of us already know that fresh juices are far more healthful than soft drinks, coffee, tea, and alcoholic beverages. But consumers may not be aware that many canned, bottled, and cartoned juices are not what they appear to be.

Did you know, for example, that Beech-Nut Nutrition Corp. was recently indicted on charges of selling millions of bottles of flavored sugar-water labeled 100-percent apple juice between 1978 and 1983? Executives of the food company allege they did not know about the phony contents of thousands of imported barrels marked "apple concentrate."

Or did you know that "Florida-Squeezed" juices may be made from fruit treated with banned pesticides? To save money, some juice manufacturers import cheap citrus fruit to the United States, where it is then *"Florida-Squeezed."* This advertising fib might be forgivable if it ended there. It does not. Consumers should be aware that imported produce—and juices made from imported produce—may carry traces of banned pesticides. Several countries that export fruits and vegetables, including Mexico, continue to use pesticides such as dichloro diphenyl trichloroethane (DDT), though the United States Environmental Protection Agency (EPA) has banned the use of DDT and several other such carcinogenic pesticides on U.S.-grown produce. (Read more about pesticides in Chapter 7.)

Other little-known juice facts center on the new "juicey" type "natural" juices. Did you know, for instance, that these are made from fruit concentrates and not whole fruit juices? Though many concentrates are of the highest quality—if not the highest nutritional value—they are only as good as the liquids with which they are reconstituted. Enter industrial water. Consumers who prefer to drink spring water, or who are sensitive to the many chemical resins found in municipally supplied water, might want to know that both imported and domestic fruit concentrates are reconstituted with filtered tap or well water from factory property in industrially zoned areas.

Finally, to this ample list of caveats, the caution on additives is attached. By now, it is common knowledge that food manufacturers routinely add artificial colors and flavors, sugar, corn syrup, salt, and chemical preservatives to their products—and juices are no different.

But are commercially manufactured juices really the bad guys of nutrition? Granted, the results of drinking less-than-fresh juices are not fatal. But by advertising their products as "natural" or "health" beverages, juice manufacturers often mislead consumers who seek to build vitality with alternatives to chemical-filled, carbonated soft drinks. At the very least it is ironic that many consumers don't realize many packaged juices are as nutritionally vapid as the soft drinks they would replace!

For those seeking more healthful alternatives, this book advocates drinking pure, fresh juices made at home with an electric juice extractor. The key word here is "fresh." For, as we recommend several high-quality bottled juices in this book (see Chapter 8), fresh juices remain the superior choice in both taste and nutrition. Just one pint of fresh carrot juice, for example, contains more than 20,000 international units (IUs) of pro-vitamin A in its purest and most natural form. That is *four times* the Recommended Daily Allowance (RDA) for vitamin A. (Read more about RDAs in Chapter 1.)

Because of their nutritional excellence, juices may prevent diet-related illnesses. A growing body of research reveals that juice may even cure a variety of illnesses and conditions, as well. For instance, cabbage juice contains vitamin U, which has been shown to heal peptic ulcers; while fresh apple and prune juices are excellent laxatives. Green juices contain enzymes that foster weight loss by stimulating the metabolic system. Alfalfa sprout juice supplies vitamin K, a blood coagulant important to the health of pregnant women. Watermelon and cucumber juices have a safe, natural diuretic action. Studies done by the National Academy of Sciences conclude that the pro-vitamin A content of orange, yellow, and green vegetable juices may help prevent some forms of cancer.

While the list of juice therapies continues to grow, it's only half the story. Granted, eliminating disease is a worthy goal, but should it be our only aim? Or, rather, should we strive with equal resolve to achieve and maintain optimal healthfulness? If we choose the latter course, we cannot ignore the effects of daily nutrition on long-term health. And although fresh juice provides excellent nutrition, it is not a "magic bullet." The maximum long-term health benefits will be achieved by incorporating fresh juices into a nutritious and balanced diet.

Unfortunately, our diets often sabotage our best health interests. Most people living in the Western world today eat too few fresh fruits and vegetables and too many overcooked, processed foods that contain excess fat and protein. To be truly healthy in this age of fast foods, environmental pollutants, and stress, many nutritionists now recommend that we get two to five times the RDA for several key vitamins and minerals. Unfortunately, many of these nutritionists prescribe the high-tech solution: synthetic multi-vitamin/mineral pills. Why is this the wrong approach?

Most vitamin/mineral pills are synthesized from coal tar or other petroleum derivatives. For this reason, while they may be chemically identical to vitamins found in foods or fresh juices, they may have only a fraction of the *biological activity* of vitamins found in live foods. Synthetic vitamins are not absorbed as well as those found naturally in foods. One laboratory study revealed that, when mixed with nonnutritive synthetic food bases, synthetic vitamins are unable to sustain human life. They are missing "something" that scientists have not been able to synthesize in their labs. That something includes live enzymes. It is called the "life force."

Compared with synthetic vitamins, naturally derived vitamins from fresh fruits, vegetables, sprouts, grasses, and their juices were designed by Nature to supply high-quality nutrition capable of sustaining human life. One pint of fresh vegetable juice, for example, supplies the same live vitamins, minerals, and enzymes found in two large vegetable salads. The human body assimilates these nutrients in minutes. If a large vegetable salad is added to this juice intake daily, along with healthy portions of lightly-cooked vegetables and plenty of whole grains, it will exceed the RDA for several key vitamins and minerals by as much as 500 percent. (We will discuss these key nutrients in Chapter 1.)

Beyond their healthfulness, fresh juices are simple to prepare. And many people agree that their uniform consistency makes them even more delicious than the fresh fruits or vegetables from which they are made. To prove it, I have included dozens of my favorite fresh juice recipes in Chapter 7. Once you try them, you'll see why juicing is such a simple good habit to develop. The conclusions on the nutritional benefits of fresh juice deserve a place with none other than the greatest health discoveries this century. You can prove this to yourself over the next few weeks. Read this book from cover to cover, purchase a juicer (the better models are reviewed in Chapter 3), and drink one or two glasses of fresh juice daily. In only a few days you will begin to look and feel better, all the time gaining valuable confidence in your ability to reach optimal health and well-being. Then you'll know firsthand the difference between juice fact and fiction.

1
Juice and Nutrition

Though advances in the natural and technological sciences have catapulted humanity forward, the science of nutrition remains at a comparative standstill. Perhaps not regarded as "high-tech" research, the study of nutrition is nonetheless equally capable of unlocking mysteries that hold men hostage to ignorance.

At present, relatively little documented research exists on the nature and importance of food enzymes or the role of digestion in disease prevention. The United States Food and Nutrition Board's Recommended Daily Allowances (RDA) are sorely in need of revision, health advocates say. More mainstream research is needed, as well, to support evidence that there are significant differences between the body's use of synthetic and natural vitamins. We will learn more about these topics and their relationship to fresh juices later in this chapter.

Debate about nutrition lies at the crossroads of health in America. The good news is that people are aware of the importance of proper nutrition. The bad news is that many consumers accept the message sent out by the $2 billion vitamin industry that poor nutrition can be counteracted by popping pills. The truth is, it cannot.

While dosing ourselves and our families with synthetic vitamin pills may appear to be a convenient way to get optimal nutrition, in reality it is an ineffective long-term choice. The fact is, virtually all of the so-called "natural" or "organic" vitamins and other nutritional supplements sold in supermarkets, pharmacies, and health food stores today are compounded of more than 90 percent *unnatural* ingredients. The 10-percent balance may have been derived from a natural source, such as a plant; but it is certainly not "organic" if it is not alive. It is precisely because synthetic supplements are manufactured from chemicals and dead food that the body does not absorb, use, or dispose of them as well as organic vitamins from fresh, "live" foods. The only way to supply our bodies with natural or organic vitamins and minerals is to eat the fresh foods that contain them.

SUPPLEMENTS MAY BE HARMFUL

But synthetic supplements are not simply undesirable because they supply inferior nutrition that the body then uses inefficiently. Prolonged use or misuse of vitamin and mineral supplements may actually hurt us more than help us. By taking too much of one supplement, we initiate a negative chain reaction that destroys the balance of all other chemical levels in our body. This does not mean that taking, say, an iron pill for a few days will cause illness. It probably won't make a difference. But, over a prolonged period, taking iron pills to treat iron-deficiency anemia may accentuate the problem.

To illustrate, let's examine in detail the body's reaction to self-treatment with high doses of synthetic iron pills. Adrenal glands are stimulated by the introduction of excess inorganic iron. As a reaction, sodium levels rise. Rising sodium causes magnesium levels to plunge. This signals calcium levels to sink, which in turn causes the potassium level to jump; which in turn decreases levels of copper and zinc. The net result is a chemical imbalance capable of producing a host of symptoms from headaches to heart palpitations. Most significant, however, this chemical balancing act depletes iron further, leaving the body more anemic than when it began.

If, on the other hand, the anemic person had eaten an abundance of fresh, iron-rich foods such as leafy green vegetables, prunes, black raspberries, and Bing cherries, the body would have absorbed all the organic iron it needed and excreted the excess. The body knows when to say "no" to iron in its natural, organic form; it can't always tell when to stop with a continuing barrage of synthetic supplements.

Now that you have seen what types of gyrations the body must perform to balance vitamin overdoses, perhaps you can understand how certain nutritionists and health professionals suspect that long-term overuse of synthetic supplements may lead to some diseases.

THE DISCOVERY OF VITAMINS

In the early 1900s, a Polish chemist named Casimar Funk developed the vitamin theory while examining the causes of four widespread diseases: beri-beri, pellagra, rickets, and scurvy. At first, Funk believed these illnesses were caused by poisons in the diets of the sufferers. However, continued research disproved this theory. By process of elimination, he concluded that elements missing from the diet were the causes of these problems.

Funk set out to identify these missing elements. By administering various natural components to diseased patients, he was able to observe their effects firsthand. He concluded that deficiencies in four specific elements were responsibile for causing the symptoms of these diseases. Funk identified vitamin B-1 deficiency as the cause of beri-beri; niacin deficiency as the cause of pellagra; vitamin D deficiency as the cause of rickets; and vitamin C deficiency as the cause of scurvy. To prove his theory, he administered the element to the patient with the corresponding deficiency and, in each case following a brief period of vitamin therapy, the disease abated.

Funk named the elements he discovered vitamins, literally, "union of vitality." His choice of this name reflects his belief that vital, uncooked, or "live" foods are important to maintain health.

THE FUNCTION OF VITAMINS

Throughout this century, scientists and nutritionists have added to the body of knowledge about vitamins. Thanks to their efforts, we now know that vitamins are organic compounds, effective in minute amounts, that the body cannot manufacture on its own. They are used as fuel to energize essential processes such as metabolism, growth, and repair. Though humans need only minuscule amounts of a broad spectrum of vitamins, a deficiency of only one can rapidly produce symptoms associated with disease.

Fresh juices are excellent sources not only of vitamins, but of a host of other important nutrients, as well. Incorporated into a balanced, whole foods diet, fresh juices will provide more than an adequate supply of vitamins and nutrients to maintain optimal health. And unlike synthetic supplements, fresh-squeezed juices will do this without danger of toxicity, buildup, or imbalance.

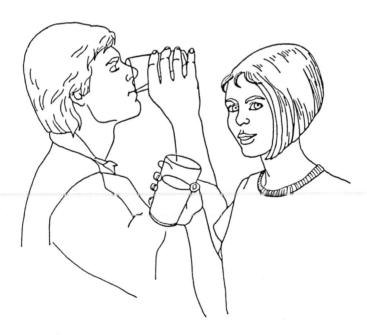

**Fresh juices are excellent sources of vitamins
and a host of other important nutrients.**

RDA, ODA, AND JUICES

As we have seen, organic vitamins and minerals are, clearly, essential to good health. But just how much is enough?

At present, within this country's medical and nutritional communities, there exist divergent opinions about the validity of the nutritional guidelines we know as the Recommended Daily Allowances (RDA). The RDAs have served as a guide for Americans to follow to achieve good nutrition for more than forty years. But growing evidence points to the possibility that RDAs may, in many cases, represent only a fraction of the actual amounts of vitamins and minerals we require. Those who cite this evidence say that the one-size-fits-all mentality behind the RDA is uneven. At best, they say, the RDA represents the "minimum wages of nutrition."

To compound this problem, many Americans aim to satisfy the RDA by eating commercially-grown, processed foods which have, in many cases, lost substantial nutrient value. The effect of seeking minimum nutrition from nutrient-deficient food sources is, quite possibly, nutritional disaster.

To resolve this problem, many nutritionists and concerned health professionals now recommend adherence to an *Optimum Daily Allowance* (ODA) guideline to achieve not minimum but optimum nutrition. For an example of how the ODA compares to the RDA, refer to Table 1.1.

A personal ODA is arrived at by weighing several factors: age; weight; family history; emotional, physical, and environmental stress. These amounts are often, although not always, in excess of the amounts found in the RDA. The important point is not that one plan exceeds another, but rather that the ODA is a *personalized* approach to nutrition.

Fresh-squeezed juices can play a major role in satisfying your ODA. Unlike processed foods that are the mainstay of many Americans' diets, they are packed with vitamins, minerals, fluids, enzymes, amino acids, and chlorophyll. We'll examine each of these nutritional components in the pages that follow. For more detailed nutrient information, you may refer to Appendix A and Appendix B.

Table 1.1 Comparison of RDA and Sample ODA Profiles

NUTRIENTS:	RDA	ODA	ODA
	Profile: All Adults.	Profile: Businessman, 35, with spastic colon; family history bowel cancer.	Profile: Retired teacher, 67, with arthritis and osteoporosis.
Vitamin A; Beta carotene	4,000-5,000 IU	10,000 IU 50,000 IU	10,000 IU 10,000 IU
Vitamin D	400 IU	400 IU	800 IU
Vitamin E	10-20 IU	800 IU	1,200 IU
B complex (B-1, B-2, B-3, B-6)	1.2-1.4 MG	50 MG	100 MG
Vitamin B-12	3 MCG	None.	None.
Folic acid	400 MCG	None.	None.
Vitamin C	60 MG	5,000 MG with 2,400 MG Bioflavonoids	5,000 MG with 5,000 MG Bioflavonoids
Calcium	800 MG	1,000 MG	2,000 MG
Phosphorus	800 MG	(from diet)	400 MG
Magnesium	300-500 MG	500 MG	1,000 MG
Zinc	15 MG	50 MG	50 MG
Iron	10-18 MG	15 MG	25 MG
Copper	None.	2 MG	2 MG
Manganese	None.	15 MG	30 MG
Chromium	None.	200 MCG GTF Chromium	200 MCG GTF Chromium
Selenium	None.	300 MCG	200 MCG
Iodine	150 MCG	50 MCG	300 MCG
Potassium, PABA, Biotin, Choline, Pantothenic acid, Inositol	None.	None.	None.

ODA data adapted from Design Your Own Vitamin and Mineral Program, Shari Lieberman, M.A., R.D., and Nancy Bruning, Doubleday & Co., 1987. RDA data published in Recommended Dietary Allowances, Food and Nutrition Board of the Institute of Medicine, National Academy of Sciences, Ninth Edition, 1980.

The above chart illustrates how different people require different amounts of nutrients. Note that the two ODA profiles match or omit nutrients in the RDA. The important point about the ODA is not that it exceeds the RDA, but that it is personalized.

VITAMINS IN FRESH JUICES

If you're looking for vitamin potency, fresh juices deliver. Just choose the vitamins you want and drink the juices that contain them. It's as simple as that.

Vitamin A (retinol) promotes normal growth and development, fosters proper eyesight, maintains clear, healthy skin, and has been linked to cancer prevention. Fresh carrot or green juices contain an abundance of *pro-vitamin A* (beta carotene). Pro-vitamin A is easily converted to usable vitamin A in the liver. Unlike synthetic vitamin A, which is toxic in high doses, pro-vitamin A from food sources is safe even in large amounts.

The *vitamin B complex* is a group of vitamins that works together to help the body digest and use the energy in carbohydrates. B complex also promotes resistance to infection.

Components of B complex are: *vitamin B-1* (thiamine), *vitamin B-2* (riboflavin), *vitamin B-3* (niacin), *vitamin B-6* (pyridoxine), *vitamin B-12* (cobalamine), *biotin, choline, folic acid, inositol, PABA,* and *pantothenic acid.* Whole grains are among the best natural sources of B complex vitamins. But fresh juices, especially green and sprout juices, and citrus juice made with a high-speed juicer contain significant amounts of B complex vitamins, as well.

Vitamin C is regarded popularly as a panacea, capable of curing colds, heart disease, cancer, and other ailments. However, the clinical evidence that vitamin C does any of these things is inconclusive. What *has* been proven is that vitamin C is an antioxidant—a substance that protects important molecules and structures in the cells from being destroyed by oxygen. It helps protect the nerves, glands, joints, and connective tissues from oxidation, and also aids in the absorption of iron. All fresh fruit and vegetable juices are excellent sources of vitamin C.

Vitamin E is another important antioxidant. It helps the heart to function, and promotes the use of fatty acids. Because studies on animals show it to be true, scientists hypothesize that vitamin E may also protect fertility in women and men. Fresh beet, celery, and green juices contain vitamin E, as do whole grains, seeds, and nuts.

MINERALS IN FRESH JUICES

Minerals found in foods are quite different from those found in supplemental mineral pills as we learned in the explanation at the beginning of this chapter. In foods, minerals are always combined with specific amino acids; sometimes with vitamins. The process of bonding mineral to amino acid or mineral to vitamin is called "chelation." Chelated minerals are preferable to synthetic minerals because the body easily recognizes and uses minerals in chelated form. This is why a diet rich in easy-to-assimilate organic minerals will help ensure the body maintains all its important minerals in proper ratio.

The balanced, chelated minerals in fresh juices help keep the body's energy level high; the nerves calm; and the muscles, heart, hair, teeth, bones, and nails strong. They also keep the blood clean and the blood pH (its relative alkalinity or acidity) balanced. They do this by neutralizing acid and alkaline ash, waste products of human digestion and metabolism.

In addition to these general functions, each mineral has a specific function. The specific functions of several of the major minerals contained in fresh juices are described below.

Potassium is responsible for the electrochemical balance of tissues of the heart and all other muscles. *Iron* is a component of red blood cells. It transports oxygen to the lungs and aids in cell respiration. *Phosphorus* is essential to the proper function of the brain and nerves. *Calcium* maintains the acid/alkaline balance of the blood and strengthens bones.

Sulfur aids the functioning of the brain and nerves. It is a body cleanser. *Iodine* fuels the thyroid gland, which controls the body's metabolism. *Magnesium* aids in muscle relaxation, protein synthesis, energy production, and is a natural laxative.

Manganese is necessary in the functions of the brain. *Germanium* aids in the function of the immune system and bowels. Studies show it may help alleviate mood disorders. *Selenium* works with vitamin E to delay oxidation of fatty acids.

Sodium, with potassium, calcium, and magnesium, works to neutralize acids, maintain cell integrity, and keep tissues' electromagnetic energy intact.

FLUIDS IN FRESH JUICES

Another valuable health property of fresh juices is their *fluid* content. At least 65 percent of the body is composed of water. Water is a major component of the blood. Blood feeds the cells and carries away waste products of metabolism. Therefore, the more healthy the blood, the more vital the cells and overall bodily health. Fresh juices help to cleanse the blood while improving its important chemical and electromagnetic qualities. They transfer live plant energy to our bodies.

Beverages such as coffee, tea, soft drinks, beer, flavored drinks, alcoholic beverages, and municipal water contain sugar, additives, preservatives, chlorine, fluoride, caffeine, and a host of other ingredients that the body must eliminate before it meets its needs for purified fluids. Key organs of elimination such as the kidneys and liver are taxed by the work necessary to expel the many foreign elements and non-nutritive substances in these beverages.

Unlike the fluid in these drinks, the fluid in fresh juices is pure water, distilled by Nature in the plant or tree. It contains no harmful substances. It does not tax the organs of elimination.

Not simply healthful, the pure fluids in fresh juices are excellent for quenching the thirst, as well. You can make a superior mineral-electrolyte drink to take after strenuous exercise by juicing four parts watermelon rind with one part each cucumber and celery, and mixing an equal proportion of this juice with spring water. Packed with minerals, this juice has a slightly salty taste.

ENZYMES IN FRESH JUICES

Enzymes are the body's labor force, the active construction-and-demolition teams that constantly build and rebuild the body. Approximately 1,000 different enzymes are known. At any one time there will be millions of enzymes working in every living body. Without enzymes a human would be a lifeless pile of unusable chemicals. Outside the human body, enzymes are found in all living things, including food in its raw, uncooked state. It is the enzymes in a green tomato, for example, that cause it to ripen and turn red.

Each food is replete with enzymes that help break down the elements found within it. For example, bananas are rich in carbohydrates and contain *amylase*, a carbohydrate-splitting enzyme. Raw butter (high in saturated fat) is rich in *lipase*, a fat-splitting enzyme. Uncooked or smoked fish or meats are rich in protein-splitting enzymes. When foods are eaten raw, the food enzymes within them do much of the work of breaking down the foods in our stomachs and small intestines, saving our bodies' own enzyme labor force from having to do so.

However, enzymes are extremely sensitive to heat. When foods are cooked, all of their helpful enzymes are destroyed, just as a prolonged fever will burn up the enzymes in the body.

I have researched the matter of food enzymes for years, and have worked with thousands of people experimenting with dietary changes to include more fresh foods. As a result, I recommend that a minimum of 25 percent of the diet be composed of raw fresh foods, such as fruits and vegetables, certified raw dairy products (available at natural foods stores), nuts and seeds (in moderation), sprouts, greens, and, of course, fresh juices.

It is more natural to eat raw foods during the warmer months when they are available locally and are plentiful. During this time an even greater amount of raw food can be eaten for the purposes of cleansing the body of winter's inactivity. Also, during the transition to eating more fresh foods, it is helpful to begin exercising more, in order to speed up metabolism. This makes digestion smoother and easier.

After cooling down from exercise, try restoring your fluid and mineral balances with a glass of fresh juice. It will feel like you have exercised your muscles with activity and your cells with fresh juice—a double workout!

In summary, fresh juices are excellent sources of important food enzymes, as are all raw foods. Even though too little is currently known about their vital role in health, by observing the positive effects they create, I am convinced that fresh foods and juices should comprise a generous portion of the diet.

AMINO ACIDS IN FRESH JUICES

Next to water, *protein* is the most plentiful element in the body. More than 50 percent of the dry weight of the body is composed of protein. Proteins, in turn, are composed of protein chains called *amino acids*. Whereas enzymes do the building, amino acids are the raw materials used to build. Together enzymes and amino acids are responsible for cell renewal and an array of diverse functions—from the making of hormones to the building of muscles, blood, and organs.

There are eight major amino acids called *essential* amino acids, which the body can synthesize only from the foods we eat. If these eight are not present in the diet, the body is unable to rejuvenate the cells properly, and deficiency symptoms will arise. In addition to these eight, there are a dozen known amino acids that are just as important—but can be formed by the body internally.

Amino acids are links that compose complex protein chains. They are involved in thousands of body functions and systems. Key among these are the proper digestion and assimilation of foods, cell renewal, immunity from disease and illness, rapid healing of wounds, and proper liver function.

A deficiency of just one amino acid can cause a range of symptoms from allergies to poor digestion to premature aging. However, the replacement of that same amino acid can just as easily result in a complete reversal of the situation. In short, the numerous essential amino acids found in fresh juices and whole natural foods can make the difference between fair health, mental sluggishness, and weak immunity and vital health, mental clarity, and strong immunity.

All fresh juices contain amino acids in an easy-to-digest form; however, those made using plenty of sprouts and leafy greens will contain the highest concentrations of essential amino acids.

Let's take a look at the eight essential amino acids found in fresh juices.

Lysine is one amino acid that received attention lately as a potential anti-aging factor. It helps to activate hormones and enzymes. Body growth and blood circulation are fostered by this important amino acid. Without enough lysine, our immune response weakens, sight may be affected, and fatigue can occur.

Leucine is an amino acid that keeps us alert and awake. In fact it is not recommended that insomniacs use this amino acid by itself as it can worsen their problem. Nevertheless, an adequate supply of leucine is necessary for anyone who wants to experience high-energy living.

Another amino acid you may have heard of, or seen listed in many vitamin-mineral formulas, is tryptophan. It is essential for building rich, red blood; healthy skin and hair. Working with the B complex vitamins, tryptophan also helps to calm the nerves and stimulate better digestion.

Other essential amino acids are phenylalanine, which aids the thyroid gland in its production of thyroxin hormone, which is necessary for mental balance and emotional calm; threonine, which stimulates smooth digestion, assimilation of foods, and overall body metabolism; and valine, which activates the brain, aids muscle coordination, and calms the nerves. A deficiency of valine may lead to nervousness, mental fatigue, emotional outbursts, and insomnia.

The last of the eight essential amino acids is methionine, which helps cleanse and regenerate cells of both the kidney and liver. It also may stimulate hair growth and mental calmness. Its effect is nearly the opposite that of leucine; methionine calms rather than excites the emotional and mental processes.

CHLOROPHYLL IN FRESH JUICES

Chlorophyll is a green, proteinous compound found in the leaves of plants and in grasses. As an external and internal healer and cleanser, fresh chlorophyll juice is second to none. In numerous laboratory and clinical trials, green juices proved to be an effective antiseptic, cell stimulator and rejuvenator, and red-blood-cell builder. Recent laboratory studies also indicate that green vegetables can help the body to prevent the formation of certain types of cancer.

In my opinion, chlorophyll—especially in the form of wheatgrass juice—is a super blood and cell builder, cleanser, and overall regenerative tonic. The chlorophyll molecule itself is remarkably similar to hemoglobin, the substance that carries oxygen in the blood. The illustration that follows details the chemical similarity between plant chlorophyll and human hemoglobin. In numerous experiments, animals have been able to convert chlorophyll into hemoglobin, thereby enriching the blood. It is believed by some health researchers that humans have the same ability.

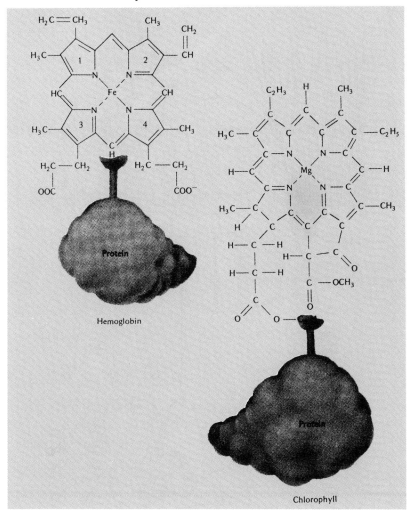

A Comparison of Chlorophyll and Hemoglobin

From *Biology: A Human Approach* by Irwin W. and Vilia G. Sherman. Copyright © 1975 by Oxford University Press, Inc. Reprinted by permission.

Fresh juices are wonderful for getting chlorophyll into the diet. Leafy greens such as lettuce, kale, collards, chard, alfalfa, cabbage, spinach, buckwheat greens, sunflower greens, turnip greens, watercress, parsley, celery, cucumbers, scallions, and green peppers are just a few of the chlorophyll-packed green vegetables that can be added to nutritious juice combinations.

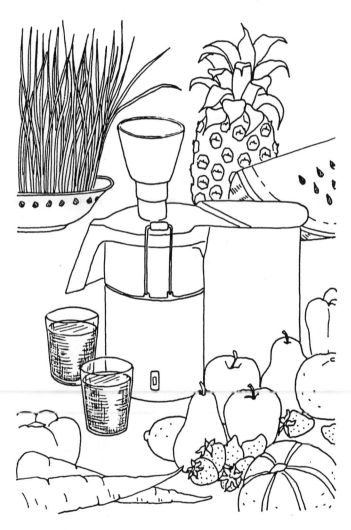

**There is virtually no limit to the variety
of fresh juices you can make.**

2

Designing a
Juice Program

A personalized juice program is simple to design and simple to follow. However, if you are not accustomed to drinking juices on a regular basis, it's best to begin slowly. Like most beginners, you may choose to embark on your juice program simply by increasing your daily intake of such juice favorites as apple, orange, tomato, or grape. Later, you may incorporate juices with specific health benefits such as wheatgrass, purslane, and kohlrabi. Though not as tasty as those listed above, these are excellent tonics for specific ailments. To help you get started, sample juice programs are listed at the end of this chapter.

While fresh juices are high in nutrition, they are low in fiber. A fiber-rich diet will complement your juice program by supplying the bulk your body needs for proper digestion. To be certain you are getting enough dietary fiber, you must eat at least two fiber-rich meals each day. Foods high in fiber include raw vegetables, whole grain cereals and breads, and whole fresh fruits. By adding fiber-rich meals to a sound juice program, you will be taking the most positive step you can toward better health.

REGIONAL PRODUCE:
THE NUTRITION CONNECTION

There are several reasons why selecting fruits, vegetables, and greens that have been grown in your region of the country will ensure you get the maximum nutrition from the fresh juice you make from them.

There is a virtual consensus in the health profession that fruits, vegetables, and greens contain peak nutrition when they are ripe. But more than 60 percent of the United States' commercially grown fruits, vegetables, and greens are picked several days *before* they are ripe. Early harvesting is common procedure in the three states responsible for growing and transporting the majority of this country's produce. These states are California, Florida, and Texas. Once harvested, much of the produce from these states is packed and shipped elsewhere. As a result, it is often days or even weeks old—yet still not naturally ripe—by the time it is displayed for sale at your local market. Modern agricultural science has introduced fungicides, coolants, and chemicals to enhance the appearance and retard the perishability of commercially grown produce. Unfortunately, it has done so at the expense of nutrition.

Regionally grown fruits, vegetables, and greens, on the other hand, don't have to be picked before they ripen because they don't have to travel far to your local market. This allows them to ripen to maturity on the vine or in the earth—ensuring that the consumer gets all the nutrition that Nature intended.

A final consideration but, by no means the least important, a vote for regional produce is a vote for your region's farming industry. By choosing regionally grown produce, you can help to ensure that your region's farms don't become parking lots and shopping malls.

WHEN TO DRINK YOUR FRESH JUICES

Most folks "bolt down" beverages of all types during meals. But this is the worst time to do so. Why? There are two reasons.

First, during the process of digestion, foods are broken down to their most useful elements to be used as fuel. Nature has given us chemically balanced saliva and digestive juices to help carry on this important process. By adding liquids to that process, we dilute and weaken the body's own digestive juices and, in turn, its digestive process.

Second, fresh juices contain highly concentrated sugars and starches. These can ferment in the digestive tract while waiting for the food eaten with them to be digested. This can result in all types of digestive upsets. For both of these reasons, it is best to drink fresh juices on an empty stomach—either one-half hour before meals, one-half hour after meals, or as between-meal snacks.

WHERE TO FIND THE BEST JUICE INGREDIENTS

Organically grown produce is the ideal choice for juicing. Naturally, a backyard garden is the best place to harvest organically grown produce. It's also the best place to harvest greens such as dandelion and lamb's-quarters. By harvesting from your own backyard, you can ensure these greens have not been affected by highway fumes or contaminated soil. Of course, you'll want to make certain that nothing you harvest from your garden, including wild greens, has been sprayed with harmful chemicals of any type—this includes those contained in many common lawn fertilizers, pesticides, and fungicides.

The next choice for organically grown produce is your local health food store. While its selection pales with the supermarket, you can be sure that produce sold here has been grown organically and/or regionally.

If you must shop for produce in supermarkets, check that you are buying organically grown and/or regionally grown produce. Several West Coast supermarket chains now carry certified organic produce. Grocery stores across America have begun to stock pesticide-free foods. To obtain a list of such stores, you may send a self-addressed, stamped envelope to: Organic Crop Improvement Association, 3185 Township Road, #179, Bellefontaine, OH 43311. Meanwhile, don't hesitate to ask the manager of your supermarket's produce department

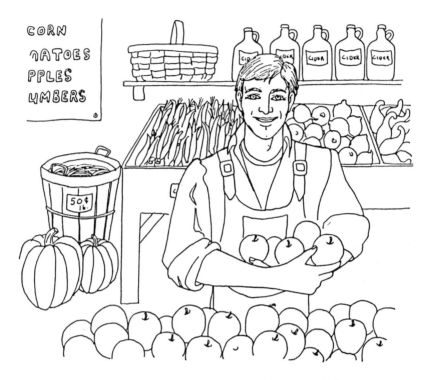

CORN
nATOES
PPLES
UMBERS

50¢
lb.

**Farmers at roadside produce stands can advise you
where to buy nutritious fruits and vegetables year-round.**

the country or state of origin of any fruit, vegetable, or green displayed for sale.

For more specific information on pesticides in commercially sold fruits and vegetables, you may contact Mothers and Others for Pesticide Limits at the Natural Resources Defense Council, Box 96641, Washington, DC 20090. For $7.95 (check or money order), they will send you their book *For Our Kids' Sake: How to Protect Your Child from Pesticides in Food.*

Good alternatives to supermarket produce are the fruits and vegetables you can find at roadside produce stands in your area during peak growing seasons when they are plentiful. Ask the farmers there when and where to buy clean produce throughout the year to be sure you're getting optimum nutrition from your fruits and vegetables and the juices you make from them.

SAMPLE JUICE PROGRAMS

The juice programs that follow are meant to be starting points. Feel free to jump off and branch out with your own program once you have found what works best for you.

Health Builder

The goal of this simple juice program is to maximize overall healthfulness. Begin by drinking one, 8-ounce glass of fruit and/or vegetable juice daily. To this, you may add one or two ounces of wheatgrass juice, either undiluted or blended with other juices.

Blood and Immune Booster

A long-term cleansing juice program, this regimen will help reduce blood toxicity levels and improve immune system function within the first two weeks of use. It consists of switching from a highly refined, low-bulk diet to a natural foods diet that includes a daily supplement of three, 8-ounce glasses of fresh juice.

Body Cleansing Fast

This brief juice fast provides the quickest path we know to cleanse the body of impurities. Detailed instructions are given in Chapter 6.

Health Restorer

A simple regimen, this restorative juice program is less focused on cleansing, more focused on slow building. It consists of adding fresh juices, one glass at a time, to the regular diet over several weeks or months. Other dietary changes should be added as they are tolerated.

Keep in mind that you alone must determine what works best for you. If your juice regimen yields no results after several weeks, you may want to consider whether it is working for you. On the other hand, if your juice regimen seems to work well after a short while, you may consider maintaining that regimen, or even increasing it. In the final analysis, determining and altering the amounts and varieties of juices in your diet to achieve optimal results is your responsibility.

3
Choosing a Juicer

To make fresh juices at home, you will need a juicer. This chapter reviews the main features of the most popular juicers.

In order to select the juicer that best fits your family's needs, it helps to know a little about how a juicer differs from a blender, how it works, and how to maintain it. When you are shopping for a juicer, it is also good to know how efficient it is, how much noise and vibration it produces, and how long you can expect it to perform under normal conditions. Price and supplier are two important considerations in choosing a juicer, as well. To help you choose the juicer that's best for your family's needs, Table 3.1 lists the manufacturers' suggested retail prices for popular juicing machines. At the end of the chapter, Table 3.2 lists several juicing machine distributors to contact for purchasing information.

JUICERS VERSUS BLENDERS

A juicer differs from a blender in both method and product.

A juicer is expressly designed to extract fluid from fibers of fruits and vegetables. It works by separating liquid from pulp. Because the leftover pulp has little nutritional value and is hard to digest, it is usually discarded.

Table 3.1 Manufacturers' Suggested Retail Prices for Selected Juicers

Model	Type	Price
Acme 5001	Centrifugal	$ 160
Acme 6001	Centrifugal	230
Champion STD	Masticating	240
Chop-Rite	Manual	85
Hippocrates Complete	Wheatgrass	400
K & K Hydraulic Juicer	Manual	590
Lifestreams Electric	Wheatgrass	260
Lifestreams Manual	Wheatgrass	65
Norwalk 250i	Masticating	1,195
Norwalk 250si	Masticating	1,295
Olympic	Centrifugal	219
Phoenix AEG	Centrifugal	110
Wheateena Convertible	Wheatgrass	320
Wheateena Standard	Wheatgrass	295

Note: All prices subject to change and published for comparison purposes only.

A blender is designed to liquify whatever is fed to it by chopping it at high speed. The relatively small quantity of fluid that is released from the fibers of blended material is mixed with a high concentration of pulp. This makes for a mushy, grainy, and unpleasant-tasting beverage.

Blenders may be used to liquify non-juiceable fruits such as banana and avocado which are then added to other juices. Blenders are also acceptable to liquify the red portion of the

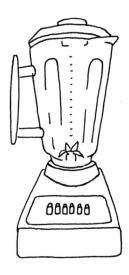

High-Speed Blender

watermelon, which is low in fiber. This liquid can be strained after blending to yield a clear juice. For day-to-day juicing, however, blenders are not recommended.

Keep in mind that while too much fiber in your juice is unpleasant, not enough fiber in your diet is unhealthy. Although fiber is low in nutrition, it is necessary for proper digestion and elimination. Because of this, fresh juices should be taken to supplement—not replace— a diet rich in high-fiber vegetables, fruits, and whole grain breads and cereals.

With this basic understanding of juicers underfoot, let's now examine in detail the various types of juicers and blenders available to today's consumers.

HIGH-SPEED JUICERS

A high-speed electric juicer is a necessity for juicing hard vegetables and fruits such as carrots, beets, apples, and celery. The four basic types of high-speed juicers are listed below:

1. **Centrifugal Juicer**. This high-speed juicer chops ("masticates") the fruit or vegetable, spins it in a plastic or stainless steel basket at high speed, and separates the juice from the pulp. The pulp remains in the basket until it is removed.

2. **Centrifugal Juicer with Pulp Ejector**. This high-speed juicer operates in the same way as the centrifugal juicer. The difference is that this version automatically ejects the pulp through a side opening.

3. **Masticating Juicer**. This high-speed juicer masticates the vegetable or fruit into a paste at high speed and then squeezes the juice through a screen in the bottom.

4. **Masticating Juicer with Hydraulic Press**. This high-speed juicer masticates the fruit or vegetable into a paste, automatically places it in a cotton bag, and hydraulically presses it.

Centrifugal Juicers

My personal favorite and one of the finest centrifugal juicers made is the Olympic Juicer. It is manufactured here in the United States and carries a ten year guarantee. It is very powerful and extracts a very high yield per pound of fruits and vegetables. It is easy to clean and recommended for juicing fruits and vegetables. The Olympic is relatively quiet and easy to operate. The juice is virtually pulp-free and requires no straining before drinking.

Other, less expensive centrifugal juicers available are the Phoenix, Braun, Oster, Sanyo, and Panasonic models. Of these five, the highest quality juices are produced by the Phoenix and the Braun. All except the Braun are small, centrifugal juicers that eject the used pulp from the machine.

All are built with smaller, less durable motors, make more noise, and are somewhat less efficient than the Olympic. However, they are a good value for the money. Manufacturers' suggested prices range from $50 to $150.

Masticating Juicers

A fine and very versatile masticating juicer is the Champion juicer. It mashes fruits and vegetables. Then it squeezes their juices from the pulp through a stainless steel screen. The Champion juicer can do double duty, serving as a grinder and blender. It grinds seeds, nuts, sprouted grains, and dried fruits to make butters, breads, and candies. And, like blenders, it can

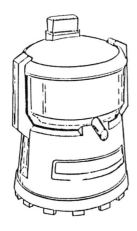

Centrifugal Juicer

be used to process frozen bananas and other fruits to make "ice cream."

The Champion comes with a five year limited warranty. Replacement parts, if they are needed, are readily available. Due to the fact that the Champion immediately ejects the pulp into a container, rather than hold it in a strainer basket, the yield of juice per pound of fruits and vegetables is considerably less than some centrifugal type juice extractors.

Another fine juicer and combination food processor, similar in capabilities to the Champion, is the Norwalk Juice Press. This unique juicer features an attached hydraulic juice press. Although the Norwalk price tag is high — approximately $1,200 — it produces the highest quality juice of all the juicers

Masticating Juicer

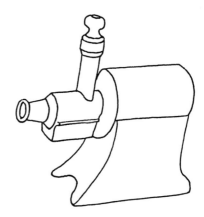

available. It is, however, large, heavy, and more difficult to carry and use than the Champion. The Norwalk is therefore recommended most often for institutional use.

JUICING BY HAND

Electric juicers fit in nicely with the pace of modern life. However, for traveling, or in the case of power failure, you may want to have a manual juicer, available in most houseware department stores, or a kit for hand-juicing. This kit might consist of an inexpensive vegetable-grating board such as a Bircher-Benner grater, and a few heavy-duty sprout or cloth bags. (You can purchase the bags from the Hippocrates Health Institute in West Palm Beach, Florida.) While this method is somewhat tiring and time-consuming, it is very efficient, and makes good juice from many different fruits and vegetables.

 To make fresh juice by hand, grate the chosen fresh fruit or vegetable finely over a bowl so that it becomes a paste. Place this paste into a sprout or cloth bag and squeeze the juice from it. Strain the juice with a fine wire mesh strainer before drinking.

WHEATGRASS JUICERS

The slow-turning juicers, often referred to as wheatgrass juicers, operate in a completely different manner than the high-speed

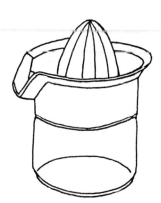

Manual Juicer

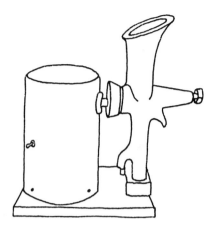

**Slow-Turning
or Wheatgrass Juicer**

juicers. The better units such as the Hippocrates or the Wheateena consist of an extra-heavy-duty motor attached to a firm base with a removable, cast-iron juicer. The motor slowly turns a blade inside the juicer, which presses the juices from leafy greens, sprouts, wheatgrass, and soft vegetables, rather than masticating them like the high-speed juicers.

Although some manufacturers claim that their high-speed juicers can extract juice from leafy greens, sprouts, and wheat-grass, they cannot do it efficiently. What little juice they do make from these delicate foods is of inferior value because high-speed processing tends to oxidize the sprout or green juices. Oxidized juice is, effectively, spoiled juice. The most obvious sign of oxidation is a grey, metallic-tasting juice.

For juicing fresh fruits or vegetables, a high-speed juicer will suffice. But if you plan to make all the recipes for juices listed in the following chapters—especially wheatgrass juice and green drinks—you will need both high- and slow-speed juicers.

WHERE TO PURCHASE A JUICER

As a rule, department stores carry a limited selection of top-of-the-line juicers. Health food stores and mail order companies are a better source for purchasing a juicer. Because they have a more specific customer base, they generally carry a wider variety of juicer models. This means the consumer gets a broader selection of models and prices from which to choose at the health food store and through the mail order company than at the department store.

By matching the model, price range, and distributor listed in this chapter to your family's needs, you will be able to choose the juicer that's right for you.

4

The Restorative Power of Fresh Vegetable and Green Juices: Alfalfa to Wheatgrass

Brimming with blood- and bone-building minerals, the fresh-squeezed juices of vegetables, sprouts, grasses, and greens have been dubbed "the body restorers." Their natural counterparts are "the body cleansers"—that is, the vitamin-packed juices of fresh fruits. In the pages that follow, you'll learn about the benefits of a variety of vegetable, sprout, grass, and green juices—from alfalfa to wheatgrass. When combined in a long-term juice therapy program, the body cleansers and the body builders can work together to achieve and maintain health.

For those who wish to read about a juice relative to a particular condition, the following chart provides information for referral. Conclusions represented by this information were arrived at after careful research, interviews with scores of health professionals, including medical doctors and nutritionists, and with other recognized experts in the fields of preventive medicine, natural foods, and nutrition. The balance of this chapter provides an overview of each vegetable listed in this chart. For further information, Appendix A correlates vitamins, minerals, bodily actions, and deficiency symptoms for vegetables commonly used to make fresh juices.

This chart should not be used in place of qualified medical advice. Only a trained physician can diagnose and treat serious and degenerative illness.

Table 4.1   Vegetable Juice Troubleshooting Chart

Condition	Recommended Vegetable Juices
Acne	Carrot, Cucumber, Dandelion Green, Endive, Fenugreek Sprout, Kohlrabi, Parsnip, Purslane, Turnip, Turnip Green, Wheatgrass
Aging (Premature)	Wheatgrass
Anemia	Alfalfa Sprout, Asparagus, Bean Sprout, Beet, Beet Green, Buckwheat Green, Dandelion Green, Endive, Kale, Kohlrabi, Lamb's-quarters, Lettuce, Parsley, Purslane, Spinach, String Bean, Swiss Chard, Turnip, Turnip Green, Watercress, Wheatgrass
Arterial Plaque	Buckwheat Green
Arthritis	Bean Sprout, Carrot, Cucumber, Fennel, Kale, Kohlrabi, Parsnip, Pepper, Sunflower Green, Turnip, Turnip Green, Wheatgrass
Asthma	Cabbage, Cabbage Sprout, Carrot, Celery, Kale, Kohlrabi, Parsnip, Radish, Radish Sprout, Scallion, Sunflower Green, Turnip, Turnip Green, Wheatgrass
Bladder Disorders	Beet, Beet Green, Cabbage, Cabbage Sprout, Carrot, Dandelion Green, Endive, Fenugreek Sprout, Kohlrabi, Parsley, Parsnip, Purslane, Sunflower Green, Summer Squash, Tomato (Fresh), Turnip, Turnip Green, Watercress, Wheatgrass

Condition	Recommended Vegetable Juices
Blood Pressure (High or Low)	Beet, Beet Green, Cabbage, Cabbage Sprout, Cucumber, Spinach, Wheatgrass
Blood Sugar Regulation (including Diabetes and Hypoglycemia)	Artichoke, Bean Sprout, Carrot, Kale, Kohlrabi, Parsnip, Spinach, String Bean, Turnip, Turnip Green, Wheatgrass
Bone Disorders (including Broken Bones)	Alfalfa Sprout, Bean Sprout, Carrot, Dandelion Green, Endive, Lamb's-quarters, Parsnip, Purslane, Tomato (Fresh), Wheatgrass
Bronchitis	Celery, Fennel, Kohlrabi, Turnip, Turnip Green, Wheatgrass
Cancer	Asparagus, Bean Sprout, Beet, Beet Green, Carrot, Kale, Kohlrabi, Parsley, Parsnip, Spinach, Sunflower Green, Swiss Chard, Turnip, Turnip Green, Wheatgrass
Cholesterol Reduction	Buckwheat Green
Circulatory Weakness	Beet, Beet Green, Buckwheat Green, Dandelion Green, Endive, Kale, Kohlrabi, Parsley, Pepper, Purslane, Spinach, Sunflower Green, Turnip, Turnip Green, Watercress, Wheatgrass
Colitis	Cabbage, Cabbage Sprout, Spinach, Wheatgrass
Constipation	Cabbage, Cabbage Sprout, Celery, Dandelion Green, Endive, Lettuce, Purslane, Spinach, Wheatgrass

Table 4.1   Vegetable Juice Troubleshooting Chart, continued

Condition	Recommended Vegetable Juices
Cough	Scallion
Eczema	Cucumber, Kohlrabi, Radish, Radish Sprout
Eye Disorders (including Cataracts and Fatigue)	Alfalfa Sprout, Asparagus, Beet, Beet Green, Carrot, Dandelion Green, Endive, Kohlrabi, Lamb's-quarters, Parsley, Parsnip, Purslane, Pepper, Sunflower Green, Turnip, Turnip Green, Wheatgrass
Fatigue	Alfalfa Sprout, Artichoke, Bean Sprout, Beet, Beet Green, Lamb's-quarters, Swiss Chard, Wheatgrass
Female Endocrine Imbalance	Parsley, Watercress
Fever	Cucumber
Fluid Retention	Bean Sprout, Cucumber, Fenugreek Sprout
Gout	Asparagus, Celery, Fennel, Tomato (Fresh)
Hair Loss	Alfalfa Sprout, Cabbage, Cabbage Sprout, Cucumber, Kale, Lamb's-quarters, Lettuce, Pepper, Watercress, Wheatgrass
Hay Fever	Carrot, Kale, Parsnip, Wheatgrass
Heart Disease	Beet, Beet Green, Buckwheat Green, Dandelion Green, Endive, Fenugreek Sprout, Kohlrabi, Parsley, Pepper, Purslane, Scallion, Spinach, Sunflower Green, Turnip, Turnip Green

Condition	Recommended Vegetable Juices
Impotence	Alfalfa Sprout, Kale, Lamb's-quarters, Wheatgrass
Infection	Kohlrabi, Scallion, Spinach, Turnip, Turnip Green, Wheatgrass
Insomnia	Celery, Lettuce
Intestinal Disorders	Watercress
Jaundice	Beet, Beet Green
Kidney Disorders	Alfalfa Sprout, Asparagus, Beet, Beet Green, Cabbage, Cabbage Sprout, Celery, Cucumber, Lamb's-quarters
Liver Disorders	Alfalfa Sprout, Beet, Beet Green, Carrot, Celery, Dandelion Green, Endive, Kale, Kohlrabi, Lamb's-quarters, Lettuce, Parsnip, Purslane, Spinach, Sunflower, Tomato (Fresh), Turnip, Turnip Green, Watercress, Wheatgrass
Lung Disorders	Kohlrabi, Sunflower Green, Turnip, Turnip Green, Wheatgrass
Lymph Circulation	Beet, Beet Green, Swiss Chard
Malnutrition	Bean Sprout
Menopause	Beet, Beet Green, Swiss Chard
Menstrual Problems	Beet, Beet Green, Swiss Chard, Watercress
Mucous Membranes (including Catarrh Elimination)	Kohlrabi, Radish, Radish Sprout, Scallion

Table 4.1   Vegetable Juice Troubleshooting Chart, continued

Condition	Recommended Vegetable Juices
Nervous Disorders	Asparagus, Celery, Fennel, Lettuce, Spinach, Wheatgrass
Poor Digestion	Spinach
Pregnancy and Delivery	Alfalfa Sprout, Bean Sprout, Beet, Beet Green, Carrot, Kale, Lamb's-quarters, Parsnip, Swiss Chard
Prostate Disorders	Asparagus, Parsley
Psoriasis	Cucumber
Pyorrhea	Cabbage, Cabbage Sprout, Kale, Spinach
Rheumatism	Asparagus
Skin Disorders	Asparagus, Beet, Beet Green, Carrot, Dandelion Green, Endive, Fenugreek Sprout, Kohlrabi, Parsley, Parsnip, Pepper, Purslane, Radish, Radish Sprout, Scallion, Spinach, String Bean, Sunflower Green, Swiss Chard, Tomato (Fresh), Turnip, Turnip Green, Watercress, Wheatgrass
Sinus Disorders	Kohlrabi, Radish, Radish Sprout
Thyroid Gland Regulation	Alfalfa Sprout, Cabbage, Cabbage Sprout, Kohlrabi, Lamb's-quarters, Radish, Radish Sprout, Spinach, String Bean, Watercress
Ulcers	Cabbage, Cabbage Sprout, Carrot, Kale, Parsnip, Spinach, Wheatgrass
Urinary Tract Infection	Parsley
Weakness (Digestive or Muscular)	Bean Sprout

Condition	Recommended Vegetable Juices
Weight Loss	Alfalfa Sprout, Artichoke, Bean Sprout, Beet, Beet Green, Buckwheat Green, Carrot, Celery, Cucumber, Dandelion Green, Endive, Fennel, Fenugreek Sprout, Kale, Kohlrabi, Lamb's-quarters, Lettuce, Parsnip, Parsley, Radish, Radish Sprout, Scallion, Spinach, Sunflower Green, Tomato (Fresh), Turnip, Turnip Green, Watercress, Wheatgrass

VEGETABLES AND GREENS: THE BODY RESTORERS

All life is based on chemical and electrical activity. Every thought, every movement, causes chemical and electrical change. If we view the human body in this way, it is easy to see how negative emotional energies such as fear and worry can bring on an ulcer; or how malnutrition from a lack of fresh, nutritious foods in the diet can cause illness. For the human body to function at optimal efficiency and achieve excellent health, it must be supplied with the basic chemicals of life. Our bodies cannot manufacture many of the chemicals we need. We can supply them in only one way: through our diets.

In this chapter on fresh vegetable and green juices, and in the next chapter on fresh fruit juices, we will discuss the roles fresh juices play in supplying and restoring vitality and health. General symptoms or conditions for which nutritionists recommend these juices are listed before each, labeled "responsive conditions." In some instances, recommendations are based on more than ten years of personal experience working with individuals. In other instances, recommendations have come from a group of noted nutritionists and pioneering health educators. This group includes Norman Walker, D.Sc., author of many fine health books, among them *Fresh Vegetable and Fruit Juices*;

H.E. Kirschner, M.D., author of *Nature's Healing Grasses* and *Live Food Juices*; Paavo Airola, international authority on nutrition and author of numerous health books; John Lust, author of *Raw Juice Therapy*; Bernard Jensen, D.C., Ph.D., health educator, author of *Foods that Heal* and *Love, Sex and Nutrition*, and founder of Hidden Valley Health Ranch in Escondido, California; Jethro Kloss, author of *Back to Eden*; Ann Wigmore, author of *The Wheatgrass Book*, *The Sprouting Book*, and *The Hippocrates Diet and Health Program*; and Laura Newman, nutritionist and author of *Make Your Juicer Your Drug Store*.

GETTING WELL NATURALLY

If we deprive our bodies of a single necessary nutrient—for example, iron, calcium, or an essential amino acid—chemical and electromagnetic imbalance in the blood, bones, and nervous system will result. The longer and more severe the deprivation, the worse the symptoms can become.

Similarly, if we take too many of the wrong kinds of nutrients into our bodies—for example, too many fats, proteins, or calories—the resulting excesses can lower the vitality of the body by blocking the flow of blood and, with it, oxygen and nutrients.

Common sense tells us that the fastest and safest route to restoring chemical imbalance, health, and energy to a diseased and tired body is to cleanse and feed the blood and cells with a full spectrum of vital nutrients.

Fortunately, Nature has provided excellent sources of these necessary nutrients in fresh fruits, vegetables, sprouts, greens, whole grains, grasses, seeds, nuts, seafood, and dairy products. Excess protein, fat, or acid wastes are stirred up and removed with the help of these nutritious, cleansing foods. Once cleansed, our cells become charged with the electromagnetic energies of these fresh foods and juices.

For nearly a century, the emphasis of health care in Western nations has been on the treatment of symptoms for which the cause is not known. Today, the focus is changing, thanks to many open-minded physicians, nutritionists, and other health care professionals. In this new view, symptoms of disease are regarded as outward signs of a general lack of balance and harmony in the sick person's life. To treat the individual, advocates of this philosophy prescribe a health-building lifestyle, rather than drugs. The purpose of this health-building lifestyle is to cleanse and strengthen the body from within. It results over the long run in freedom from all symptoms. The premise behind the health-building lifestyle is that, given the right fuel and care, the body is capable of throwing off potentially dangerous disease in its early stages. Many "miracle cures" are nothing more than the result of strict and long-term adherence to the health-building lifestyle.

For instance, in her book, *How I Conquered Cancer Naturally*, author Edyie Mae Hunsberger testified that by switching from a diet laden with sugar, salt, refined flour, and processed foods to one of live, whole natural foods, the course of her disease was reversed.

While Edyie Mae's case history does not represent adequate scientific proof in itself, her experience and that of many others has given us observable evidence that a nutritious diet will both cleanse and strengthen the body when it is combined with proper rest and exercise. A stronger, cleaner system can better defend itself against the millions of germs, stresses, and potential carcinogens we are exposed to daily. This philosophy forms the basis of the natural foods revolution.

By drinking nutritious fresh fruit and vegetable juices, you will be taking an important step on the path to symptom-free living through a health-building lifestyle.

VARIETY IS KEY

Now that we know the context within which juices are linked to health, we are ready to learn more about them. Both this chapter and the next will give you an idea of the variety of vegetables and fruits that are available for juicing. This variety itself may actually be the best protection against nutritional deficiency, because vegetables and fruits grown in different types of soils throughout the country contain different ratios of key nutrients. By increasing the variety of vegetables, fruits, and other whole, natural foods we eat, we will be less likely to develop nutritional deficiencies.

Beginning with alfalfa sprout juice, let's look at the specific health benefits supplied by some of the most beneficial fresh vegetable juices—from alfalfa to wheatgrass.

Alfalfa Sprout Juice

The king of sprouts, alfalfa is one of the most valuable plants on earth. Fully grown, its roots reach thirty feet or more into the soil, improving its fertility and drawing upon its life-giving storehouse of trace mineral elements. Most of the alfalfa grown in the United States is fed to livestock. Some is also grown for seed to make sprouts.

Alfalfa sprout juice contains valuable minerals such as calcium, chlorine, magnesium, phosphorus, potassium, silicon, sodium, and zinc, among others. Alfalfa sprout juice also supplies a full range of vitamins from A, B complex, C, and E, to vitamin K, a blood coagulant. When placed in indirect light for a couple of days before harvesting, alfalfa sprouts turn green and become a good source of nutritious chlorophyll. Alfalfa sprouts are also an excellent source of amino acids. Alfalfa sprout juice mixes well with all vegetable juices.

The best way to obtain alfalfa sprouts is to grow your own at home from organic alfalfa seed. For complete sprouting instructions, see *The Sprouting Book* by Ann Wigmore.

Selection

Choose fresh sprouts with small green leaves and keep refrigerated in plastic bag or container.

Yield

Two to four ounces juice per half pound of alfalfa sprouts.

Responsive Conditions

- Anemia
- Broken Bones
- Eye Disorders
- Fatigue
- Hair Loss
- Impotence

- Liver Disorders
- Kidney Disorders
- Pregnancy and Delivery
- Thyroid Gland Regulation
- Weight Loss

Artichoke Juice
(Jerusalem Variety)

The Jerusalem artichoke is a potato-like vegetable with a top that grows like a sunflower. It has the texture of a Chinese water chestnut without the starchiness of the potato. This makes it perfect for juicing. An analysis of the Jerusalem artichoke's chemical makeup reveals that it is an excellent vegetable source of non-starchy carbohydrates and insulin. For this reason, holistic practitioners such as Edward Cayce recommend Jerusalem artichokes for diabetic, hypoglycemic, and weight reduction diets. This vegetable reduces the craving for sweets.

You can purchase Jerusalem artichokes at the supermarket or grow your own at home as you would grow a potato. Once you plant them, they will grow and spread indefinitely. It is best to mix this juice with other sprout and vegetable juices as it tastes like potato juice by itself. It is recommended that you mix a maximum of one to two ounces of Jerusalem artichoke juice with other juices to yield an average six- to eight-ounce serving.

Selection

Choose firm artichokes with undamaged skin.

Yield

Six to eight ounces juice per pound of artichokes.

Responsive Conditions

- Diabetes
- Fatigue
- Hypoglycemia
- Weight Loss

Asparagus Juice

After the more heavy eating of winter, Nature provides spring's greens, shoots (such as asparagus), and berries to cleanse our systems of stored waste. In the spring, when the asparagus is inexpensive and plentiful here in the Northeast, I like to juice the tough stems and eat the tender tips in salads. Asparagus is a highly alkaline food. It contains the alkaloid asparagine, which reduces acidity of the blood and cleanses the tissues and muscles of waste. It helps to dissolve kidney stones.

Asparagus juice is a safe and effective diuretic. According to juice authority Norman Walker, D.Sc., asparagus juice also helps break up oxalic acid crystals imbedded in our kidneys and muscles from eating chocolate and too many cooked foods rich in oxalic acid, such as spinach and tomatoes. (Eaten raw, however, these same vegetables contain only trace amounts of oxalic acid.)

Asparagus juice is high in vitamins A, B-1 (thiamine), C, choline, folic acid, and the mineral potassium. It is an especially good addition to combinations of juices made from greens, sprouts, and vegetables.

Selection

Choose either young and firm or larger but tender asparagus. Asparagus is available across the U.S. from April through June.

Yield

One ounce juice per three to four asparagus shoots.

Responsive Conditions

- Anemia
- Cancer
- Eye Disorders
- Gout
- Kidney Disorders

- Nervous Disorders
- Prostate Disorders
- Rheumatism
- Skin Disorders

Bean Sprout Juice

Aduki, mung, and lentil beans all yield excellent sprout juice. They are rich in high quality protein. Bean sprout juice is especially good as a blood builder. Lentil sprouts, for example, are an excellent source of the mineral iron. All bean sprouts are rich in vitamin C, and when vitamin C is present with iron, the body absorbs more iron than it would without the vitamin C. Therefore, an excellent source of both vitamin C and iron would be found in lentil sprout juice.

Bean sprout juices mix well with other green and sprout juices, and especially well with vegetable juices. They can be used as a component of green drinks, as well.

Selection

Choose bean sprouts with clean, white shoots and no leaves. Mix a handful into vegetable or green juice, as it tastes unpleasant by itself.

Yield

Three to four ounces juice per pound of bean sprouts.

Responsive Conditions

- Anemia
- Arthritis
- Broken Bones
- Cancer
- Diabetes
- Fatigue

- Fluid Retention
- Malnutrition
- Pregnancy
- Weakness (Digestive or Muscular)
- Weight Loss

Beet and Beet Green Juice

Beets and beet greens are both powerful cleansers and builders of the blood. Beet green juice contains an abundance of chlorophyll, vitamins A and C, and alkaline minerals such as calcium and potassium. Beet juice is also an excellent source of vitamin B-6; the minerals choline, iron, organic sodium, and potassium; and natural sugars. And while the actual content of iron in beet roots is not as high as in some other foods, it is high-quality iron that is easily and efficiently used by the body. Iron is a builder of red blood corpuscles. Together beet root and beet green juice constitute a valuable aid in building the red blood cell count, in liver and gall bladder problems, and in menstrual and menopausal disturbances.

Since beet roots and greens are powerful kidney and blood cleansers, they should be used moderately. An ounce or two of beet juice mixed with other juices is plenty. Fresh beet juice mixes especially well with apple, carrot, and cucumber juices.

Selection

Choose firm roots of medium to large size. Trim tops. Clean and juice separately, and clean off any sand or soil before juicing. Caution: beet juice taken in excess can cause stomach upset.

Yield

Six to eight ounces juice per pound of beets or beet greens.

Responsive Conditions

- Anemia
- Bladder Disorders
- Cancer
- Circulatory Weakness
- Eye Fatigue
- Fatigue
- Heart Disease
- High Blood Pressure
- Jaundice
- Kidney Disorders
- Liver Disorders
- Low Blood Pressure
- Lymph Circulation
- Menstrual Problems
- Menopause
- Skin Disorders
- Weight Loss

Buckwheat Green Juice

Buckwheat greens are seven-day-old greens grown from whole, unhulled buckwheat seeds in one inch of soil. Mature buckwheat greens reach about eight inches in height, with pink-colored stems and round, green leaves. They taste like store-bought lettuce, yet are more nutritous and fresh, since you harvest them as needed. Though they are easy to grow at home, buckwheat greens are also available in some markets and health food stores.

Buckwheat greens are a wonderful building and cleansing food containing vitamins B-1, B-2, B-6, B-12, C, niacin, pantothenic acid; many minerals; and rutin, a natural longevity agent due to its antioxidant properties. Buckwheat greens are especially helpful in circulatory and heart problems as they also contain lecithin, a natural cholesterol-lowering fatty acid. Buckwheat juice is best mixed with other sprout, green, and vegetable juices to make green drinks.

For detailed instructions on how to grow your own buckwheat greens for just pennies a day, refer to *The Sprouting Book* by Ann Wigmore.

Selection

Choose fresh buckwheat greens with dark green leaves. Use the stems and leaves.

Yield

Six ounces juice per pound of buckwheat greens.

Responsive Conditions

- Anemia
- Arterial Plaque
- Cholesterol Reduction
- Circulatory Weakness
- Heart Disease
- High Blood Pressure
- Weight Loss

Cabbage and Cabbage Sprout Juice

Green and red cabbage and members of the cabbage family, such as Brussels sprouts, Chinese cabbage, collard greens, kale greens, and so on, are highly cleansing due to their concentration of vitamins B-6 and C (and large stores of vitamin A and calcium in kale and collard greens), and minerals including chlorine, iodine, potassium, and sulfur. Cabbage was considered to be a tonic and rejuvenator by the ancient Greeks, who also used it as a cure for baldness. Though I've never seen cabbage juice cure baldness, I have noticed that cabbage juice is an effective laxative and skin food as well as an effective healing agent for intestinal ulcers. Scientists believe the active ingredient in cabbage juice that helps heal ulcers is vitamin U.

As wonderful and valuable a cleanser and healer cabbage juice is, it may produce gas in some people. The sulfur in cabbage juice can react with bacteria in the intestines, causing mild intestinal cramping and gas. If you experience these symptoms after drinking cabbage juice, try reducing the amount used by diluting it with other juices or spring water. You may also try cabbage sprout juice rather than whole cabbage juice.

Cabbage sprouts from red, green, or Chinese cabbage seed make an equally good juice, especially when mixed with other vegetable juices.

Selection

Choose fresh, heavy heads of cabbage with green leaves. Choose fresh sprouts with green leaves.

Yield

Six ounces juice per pound of cabbage or cabbage sprouts.

Responsive Conditions

- Asthma
- Bladder Disorders
- Bronchitis
- Colitis
- Constipation
- Hair Loss

- High Blood Pressure
- Kidney Disorders
- Pyrorrhea
- Skin Problems
- Thyroid Gland Regulation
- Ulcers

Carrot Juice

Carrot juice is the king of the vegetable juices. Extremely high in pro-vitamin A, which the body converts to vitamin A, it also contains vitamins B, C, D, E, and K; as well as the minerals calcium, phosphorous, potassium, sodium, and trace minerals.

The alkaline minerals, especially calcium and magnesium, contained in carrot juice help soothe and tone the intestinal walls. At the same time, these minerals help to strengthen bones and teeth. Skin, hair, and nails benefit from its high protein and mineral content. Fresh carrot juice stimulates digestion and has a mild diuretic effect. But perhaps its most important contribution to body health is in its tonic and cleansing effect on the liver. Through regular use, carrot juice helps the liver to release stale bile and excess fats. When fat levels are reduced, cholesterol levels are reduced.

If you have heard the tale you will turn orange if you drink carrot juice, take heart. There is no such thing as a toxic dose of carrot juice. While it is true that it is possible to "overdose" on vitamin A, it is impossible to overdose on pro-vitamin A—the precursor to vitamin A that is found in abundance in carrot juice. Pro-vitamin A is converted to vitamin A in the body. It is true that drinking more than five glasses of carrot juice per week may cause the skin to yellow slightly. This is simply a manifestation of the toxins that the liver is excreting. To reduce these effects, simply decrease your dose of carrot juice. One good way to do this is to dilute your carrot juice by mixing it with other fruit and vegetable juices.

Mixed with other juices, especially sprout and green juices, carrot juice acts as a balancing element. It adds a delicious, sweet flavor to juice combinations and increases both their digestability and nutritional value. As an overall tonic and rejuvenator, carrot juice can't be beat.

Selection

Choose firm, large carrots with deep orange color.

Yield

Six to eight ounces juice per pound of carrots.

Responsive Conditions

- Acne
- Arthritis
- Asthma
- Bladder Problems
- Bone Problems
- Cancer
- Cataracts
- Diabetes

- Eye Disorders
- Hay Fever
- Liver Disorders
- Pregnancy and Delivery
- Skin Disorders
- Ulcers
- Weakness (Digestive and Muscular)
- Weight Loss

Celery Juice

Celery juice has a calming effect on the nervous system. This is probably due to its high concentration of organic alkaline minerals, especially sodium. The minerals contained in celery juice make the body's use of calcium more effective, balancing the blood's pH.

Organic sodium, which is abundant in celery juice, has received a bad name lately because of the average American's habitual overuse of inorganic sodium chloride—table salt. Unlike inorganic sodium chloride, organic sodium found in celery juice is naturally blended with many other useful minerals. It is essential to the proper functioning of all major body systems. Organic sodium is the element in blood that makes it salty.

Because of its slightly salty taste, celery juice is an excellent component of any vegetable juice combination. Celery juice is especially effective for nervous conditions because it produces a calming effect; and for weight-reduction diets, as it curbs the desire for sweets.

Selection

Choose celery that is firm and crisp. Even the greenest and toughest leaves of celery can be used to make juice. Celery juice tastes salty, and adds an excellent flavor to mixed juice drinks.

Yield

One ounce juice per two to three celery stalks.

Responsive Conditions

- Asthma
- Bronchitis
- Constipation
- Fluid Retention
- Gout

- Insomnia
- Kidney Disorders
- Liver Disorders
- Nervous Disorders
- Weight Loss

Cucumber Juice

On visits to Afghanistan, Iran, Pakistan, and Turkey, I was impressed with the popularity of the cucumber. In these countries, fresh raw cucumbers are eaten throughout the day. Street vendors peel and quarter them for a nickle. Like those around me during those sweltering days, I relied on cucumbers to supply pure liquid to help my body cool itself off.

The cucumber is a natural diuretic. It is helpful in dissolving kidney stones. It is exceptionally rich in potassium, the "youth mineral," which promotes flexibility in the muscles and gives elasticity to the cells that compose the skin. This results in a rejuvenation of the skin and facial appearance. Smart beauticians know this—and many salons include the cucumber as part of a professional facial for this reason. Cucumber juice is also a good source of silicon, sulfur, and trace elements, making it a beautifier of the hair and nails.

In their unwaxed, unpeeled form, cucumbers provide about 250 mg. of vitamin A per pound. However, it is important to note that peeled cucumbers provide virtually no vitamin A. This is because a high percentage of the vitamin A in cucumbers is concentrated in the skin. Unpeeled, waxed cukes should not be juiced because their wax will enter the juice. Rinsing the cuke in water will not remove the wax; neither will most soaps.

Therefore, it is best to peel the cukes and depend on other vegetables to provide vitamin A. For instance, why not add a carrot to your cucumber juice? By doing so, you'll add 10,000 IU of pro-vitamin A, which your body will safely convert to vitamin A.

Selection

Choose unwaxed, uniformly firm, dark green cucumbers from five to seven inches in length. Peel waxed cucumbers before juicing.

Yield

Four to six ounces juice per pound of unpeeled cucumber. Peeled cucumber yield is slightly lower.

Responsive Conditions

- Acne
- Arthritis
- Eczema
- Fever
- Fluid Retention

- Hair Loss
- High Blood Pressure
- Kidney Disorders
- Psoriasis
- Weight Loss

Dandelion Green Juice

Considered by most people to be weeds that taint a well-land-scaped lawn, dandelions make a beneficial spring tonic. The young leaves of the dandelion picked early in the spring are best. Because the tender young leaves have a slightly bitter flavor, they are best mixed with other vegetable and green juices.

Dandelion juice is exceptionally high in vitamins A and B-1 (thiamine); in minerals; and in important trace elements. It is a powerful cleanser. The potent store of vitamin A in dandelion juice makes it especially valuable as a liver cleanser and normalizer. Like carrot juice, it helps to improve eyesight and prevent night blindness. Dandelion juice is high in the minerals calcium, iron, potassium, and sodium. It contains more magnesium than garden vegetables, making it a potent alkalizer of the blood. Alkalization of the blood is especially important in the spring, when our bodies are more likely to be overly acidic due to the lack of exercise and more heavy eating of the cooler months that most likely preceded.

Magnesium, found in abundance in dandelion juice, is soothing and strengthening to the bowel wall, and to the entire muscular and skeletal structure. Magnesium combines with calcium to give strength to the bones and teeth.

Selection

Pick tender young leaves only; mature leaves are quite bitter. Avoid leaves of dandelions sprayed with weed killers or commercial fertilizers, those grown in areas close to highway fumes, or those grown in soil that contains leeched wastes from nearby dumping grounds.

Yield

One ounce juice per four to five dandelion leaves.

Responsive Conditions

- Acne
- Anemia
- Bladder Disorders
- Bone Disorders
- Circulatory Weakness
- Constipation
- Eye Disorders
- Heart Disease
- Kidney Disorders
- Liver Disorders
- Skin Disorders
- Weight Loss

Endive Juice

In some markets, this curly, lettuce-like green vegetable might also be listed under the name *escarole*. Endive is a bitter-tasting, leafy green salad vegetable that makes a juice resembling dandelion in flavor and nutritional benefit. Like dandelion, endive is best mixed with other vegetable, sprout, and green juices.

Selection

Choose fresh, firm heads. Because endive is bitter, use small amounts mixed with other vegetable juices.

Yield

Four to six ounces juice per pound of endive.

Responsive Conditions

- Acne
- Anemia
- Bladder Disorders
- Bone Disorders
- Circulatory Weakness
- Constipation
- Eye Disorders
- Heart Disease
- Kidney Disorders
- Liver Disorders
- Skin Disorders
- Weight Loss

Fennel Juice

Two varieties of fennel can be found in most supermarkets: garden fennel, used mostly as a seasoning, and florence fennel, sold fresh and resembling celery but with a sweeter taste. Florence fennel is used for juicing. It has an aroma of anise. Prepare and juice fennel as you would celery, mixing it with other green, sprout, and vegetable juice. It adds a pleasant aroma and flavor to ordinary juice combinations.

Fennel juice is nutritionally similar to celery (it is rich in alkaline minerals), though it is lower in sodium, and higher in energy-producing sugars. Due to its high calcium and magnesium content, fennel juice is especially helpful in relaxing and calming the nerves. Try a taste before bedtime instead of a glass of milk to help you wind down from a busy day. It will produce the similar calming effect without the fat and cholesterol.

Selection

Choose firm, fresh stalks of florence fennel.

Yield

Six to eight ounces juice per pound of florence fennel.

Responsive Conditions

- Arthritis
- Bronchitis
- Gout
- Kidney Troubles
- Nervous Disorders
- Weight Loss

Fenugreek Sprout Juice

Fenugreek tea is used in the Middle East as a blood builder and cleanser. It is also well known as a diuretic and cleanser of the kidneys and bladder. Fenugreek sprout juice has many of the same properties. The spicy flavor of juiced three-day-old fenugreek sprouts adds zip to combination vegetable juices. Fenugreek sprout juice is rich in a variety of minerals, including iron, phosphorus, and trace elements. Purchase seeds to grow your own fenugreek sprouts at your local health food store. For complete instructions in sprouting all types of seeds, refer to *The Sprouting Book* by Ann Wigmore.

Selection

Grow your own fenugreek sprouts. Harvest in three to five days.

Yield

Four ounces juice per pound of fenugreek sprouts.

Responsive Conditions

- Acne
- Bladder Disorders
- Fluid Retention
- Heart Disease
- Kidney Disorders
- Skin Disorders
- Weight Loss

Kale Juice

Though kale is a member of the cabbage family, its exceptionally high calcium, chlorophyll, and vitamin A content deserve special mention in a separate entry. Curly kale greens are hardy in fall and spring. They taste like cabbage and are packed with blood-building iron. The potent mixture of nutrients found in kale makes its juice especially beneficial to eyesight, bones, teeth, blood, and lymph glands, which swell if they are calcium-deficient. Kale is sold in supermarkets year-round.

Kale's high chlorophyll content helps increase the oxygen and red cell content of the blood, improving circulation and cell respiration as a result. Ounce for ounce, kale juice contains as much usable calcium as milk without milk's fat or cholesterol.

Selection

Choose fresh, firm leaves of kale.

Yield

Six ounces juice per pound of kale. Strong tasting on its own, kale juice is best blended in combination with other green, vegetable, and sprout drinks.

Responsive Conditions

- Anemia
- Asthma
- Arthritis
- Cancer
- Circulatory Weakness
- Diabetes
- Eye Disorders
- Hair Loss

- Hay Fever
- Impotence
- Liver Disorders
- Pregnancy and Delivery
- Pyorrhea
- Skin Disorders
- Ulcers
- Weight Loss

Kohlrabi Juice

Kohlrabi is a green vegetable that resembles a turnip, except that it grows above the ground. It tastes like a cross between cabbage, radish, and turnip. Strong tasting on its own, kohlrabi makes a wonderful juice for mixing with other green, sprout, and vegetable juices. Nutritionally, it is a good source of minerals such as calcium and iron. It contains other important nutrients such as carbohydrates, chlorophyll, and vitamin C.

Selection

Choose firm, fresh roots of kohlrabi.

Yield

Six to eight ounces juice per pound of kohlrabi.

Responsive Conditions

- Asthma
- Eczema
- Lung Disorders
- Mucous Membranes (including Catarrh Elimination)
- Skin Disorders
- Sinus Disorders
- Thyroid Disorders
- Weight Loss

Lamb's-Quarters Juice

Lamb's-quarters is a common weed that is very mild in flavor and rich in minerals. You can find it thriving on roadsides, in fields—almost anywhere things are growing. Though plentiful, lamb's-quarters should be picked from a place that is relatively free of auto pollution, pesticides, or soil contaminated with hazardous waste. Providing you don't spray your lawn with poisonous weed killers, your own backyard may be the best spot to harvest lamb's-quarters.

This hardy green plant with pointed leaves and tough stem may be harvested from early spring to late summer. Like alfalfa, lamb's-quarters is a deep-rooted plant that pulls trace elements up from the earth. This makes lamb's-quarters more potent in vitamins, minerals, trace elements, and enzymes than green plants with shorter roots. Lamb's-quarters juice is an overall body cleanser and builder. Juice it in combination with other greens, edible weeds, sprouts, and vegetables.

Selection

Choose fresh, green leaves grown in uncontaminated areas.

Yield

Four to six ounces juice per pound of lamb's-quarters.

Responsive Conditions

- Anemia
- Broken Bones
- Eye Disorders
- Fatigue
- Hair Loss
- Impotence

- Liver Disorders
- Kidney Disorders
- Pregnancy and Delivery
- Thyroid Gland Regulation
- Weight Loss

Lettuce Juice

Lettuce juice is both tasty and nutritious. Dark green types such as Romaine, Buttercrunch, or Bibb lettuce are the most nutritious. Head, Iceberg, Red, and Black-Seeded varieties are also good. Deep green lettuce is an excellent source of calcium, chlorophyll, iron, magnesium, potassium, silicon, and vitamins A and E. It is especially useful in rebuilding hemoglobin in the blood. Lettuce juice adds shine, thickness, and health to the hair and skin. It does more to promote hair growth than hair dressings or scalp treatments because it stimulates growth by sending vital nutrients to the roots of the hairs. Its silicon content also promotes flexibility of the muscles and joints. Iceberg lettuce in particular contains natural opiates which have a mild sedative effect, calming the nerves and relaxing the muscles.

Lettuce juice tastes rather strong undiluted. It is best mixed with other green, sprout, and vegetable juices. Use the dark green types often.

Selection

Choose fresh, heavy heads with dark green outer leaves.

Yield

Two to eight ounces juice per pound of lettuce, depending on the variety you choose. Heavy varieties yield more juice; drier, looser-leafed varieties yield less juice.

Responsive Conditions

- Anemia
- Liver Disorders
- Constipation
- Nervous Disorders
- Hair Loss
- Weight Loss
- Insomnia

Parsley Juice

The value of fresh parsley juice lies in its content of chlorophyll, vitamins (especially A and C), and minerals such as calcium, magnesium, phosphorus, potassium, sodium, and sulfur.

Aside from being nutritionally potent, parsley juice is a top-notch blood and body cleanser. It is especially helpful in cleansing the kidneys, liver, and urinary tract, due to its mix of vitamins, minerals, and chlorophyll. An excellent source of pro-vitamin A, parsley juice provides nutrients important to good eyesight. Its supplies of chlorophyll stimulate oxygen metabolism as well as cell respiration and regeneration.

Like the juice made from wheatgrass or beets, parsley juice is very concentrated, and is therefore best mixed with other vegetable and green juices. One ounce of parsley juice mixed with seven ounces of another juice or blend of juices is plenty.

Selection

Choose fresh, deep green parsley.

Yield

One to two ounces juice per three-inch bunch of parsley.

Responsive Conditions

- Anemia
- Arthritis
- Bladder Disorders
- Cancer
- Circulatory Weakness
- Eye Disorders
- Female Endocrine Imbalance

- Heart Disease
- Kidney Disorders
- Liver Disorders
- Prostate Disorders
- Skin Disorders
- Urinary Tract Infection
- Weight Loss

Parsnip Juice

The parsnip is a cream-colored, carrot-like root vegetable available at most food markets. Like carrots, parsnips are sweet and add to the flavor of other juices. Parsnips are a good source of vitamin C, chlorine, phosphorus, potassium, silicon, and sulfur, making them an important supplement to the nutrition of the skin, hair, and nails. Because it has a strong flavor, the best way to use parsnip juice is in combination with other green, sprout, and vegetable juices.

Selection

Choose large, firm roots.

Yield

Four to six ounces juice per pound of parsnips.

Responsive Conditions

- Acne
- Arthritis
- Asthma

- Eye Disorders
- Hay Fever
- Liver Disorders

- Bladder Problems
- Bone Problems
- Cancer
- Cataracts
- Diabetes

- Pregnancy and Delivery
- Skin Disorders
- Ulcers
- Weakness (Digestive and Muscular)
- Weight Loss

Purslane Juice

Purslane is a common garden weed. It grows abundantly in many areas of the world, especially during warm weather. Purslane is characterized by its low, vine-like growth and gelatinous texture. Its taste is a cross between celery, okra, and escarole, and is salty and bitter. Like other edible wild plants, purslane is both strong in flavor and concentrated in vitamins and minerals. Like most bitter foods and medicines, purslane juice stimulates the heart and circulation. It is, however, more of a cleanser than a builder of health, and those using this juice should modify their intake because of this. The mineral content of purslane juice aids the body in maintaining proper fluid balance.

Gather purslane that has grown away from well-traveled roads or other contaminated areas. Also, limit the amount of purslane juice used at one time to one ounce, mixing it well with other juices. Used moderately during warmer times of the year, it will cool and strengthen the body.

Selection

Pick purslane in the early morning, before the sun drives the liquids into the roots. Choose dark green leaves.

Yield

Two to four ounces juice per pound of purslane.

Responsive Conditions

- Acne
- Anemia
- Bladder Disorders
- Bone Disorders
- Circulatory Weakness
- Constipation

- Eye Disorders
- Heart Disease
- Kidney Disorders
- Liver Disorders
- Skin Disorders
- Weight Loss

Radish and Radish Sprout Juice

Radishes and radish sprouts, though pungent, are rich in vitamin C, iron, magnesium, and potassium. When used moderately, radish juice is both cleansing and soothing to the entire body, especially the mucous membranes located in the nasal sinuses and along the gastrointestinal tract.

Radish and radish sprout juice should always be mixed with other vegetable and green juices. A handful of radishes or radish sprouts run through the juicer per glass of mixed vegetable juice is plenty.

Selection

Select fresh-looking red radishes and radish sprouts with green leaves.

Yield

Two to four ounces juice per pound of radishes or radish sprouts.

Responsive Conditions

- Asthma
- Eczema
- Lung Disorders

- Skin Problems
- Sinus Disorders
- Thyroid Disorders

- Mucous Membranes
  (including
  Catarrh Elimination)
- Weight Loss

Scallion Juice

Like other pungent-flavored juices, scallion or green onion juice is highly cleansing to the mucous membranes of the lungs, sinuses, and digestive tract. It also stimulates the circulatory system and heart, and improves digestion and appetite. It is best to use small quantities of scallion juice, using not more than one medium scallion per glass of juice. A small scallion added to vegetable juice gives it a rich flavor and warms the body.

Selection

Choose firm, deep green scallions.

Yield

Two to three ounces juice per pound of scallions.

Responsive Conditions

- Asthma
- Cough
- Heart Disease
- Infection
- Mucous Membranes (including
  Catarrh Elimination)
- Nervous Disorders
- Skin Disease
- Weight Loss

Spinach Juice

This old standby, which brought surges of strength to the cartoon character, Popeye, is an amazingly potent cleanser and builder of the body—not, as Popeye preferred, from a can but, rather, fresh-picked.

Spinach juice is an excellent source of chlorophyll. It is also a good source of vitamins A, B complex, calcium, iron, magnesium, phosphorus, potassium, sodium, and trace elements. Its cleansing and building properties stimulate and tone the liver, gall bladder, blood and lymph circulation, and large intestine. Spinach juice has a mild laxative effect when an ounce of it is consumed along with other fresh vegetable, green, or sprout juices.

Spinach juice is especially strengthening to the teeth and gums because of its high concentration of alkaline minerals. However, because it is rich in oxalic acid (an acid that requires exercise to be metabolized), spinach juice is best used in moderate amounts, in combination with other juices, once or twice weekly. If you choose to drink more than this amount, remember to increase your activity level to compensate.

Selection

Choose firm, deep green colored spinach leaves.

Yield

Four to six ounces juice per pound of spinach.

Responsive Conditions

• Anemia	• Kidney Disorders
• Cancer	• Liver Disorders
• Circulatory Weakness	• Nervous Diseases
• Colitis	• Pyorrhea
• Constipation	• Skin Disorders
• Diabetes	• Poor Digestion
• Eye Disorders	• Thyroid Gland Regulation

- Heart Disease
- High Blood Pressure
- Infection

- Ulcers
- Weight Loss

String Bean Juice

Though you may never have thought of juicing string beans, they make wonderful juice. String bean juice is rich in B vitamins, calcium, magnesium, phosphorus, potassium, protein, and sulfur, making it valuable to the health of the skin, hair, nails, and overall metabolism of the body.

In *Fresh Vegetable and Fruit Juices*, author Norman Walker, D.Sc., mentions string bean juice as being especially helpful to diabetics, as it furnishes many of the important elements needed by the pancreas to produce insulin. It is best to use string bean juice in combination with other sprout, green, and vegetable juices because this juice tastes rather bland and has a rather gooey consistency on its own. All varieties of string beans may be juiced, although the green varieties contain more chlorophyll.

Selection

Choose firm, fresh beans. Juice, strings and all.

Yield

Four to six ounces juice per pound of string beans.

Responsive Conditions

- Anemia
- Diabetes
- Hypoglycemia

- Skin Disorders
- Thyroid Gland Regulation
- Weight Loss

Summer Squash Juice

Though summer squash varieties such as zucchini and yellow squash are not overly juicy, they make plenty of juice when put through a juicer. Summer squash juice is rich in vitamins B-1, B-2, and niacin; and rich in the alkaline minerals calcium and potassium. Drunk on a regular basis during the summer months, this juice helps to cool, soothe, and cleanse the body. Summer squash juice is best used in combination with other juices. By itself, it is quite bland tasting.

Selection

Choose firm, shiny squash.

Yield

Four to six ounces juice per pound of summer squash.

Responsive Conditions

- Bladder Disorders
- Kidney Disorders

Sunflower Green Juice

As was mentioned in the preceding discussion of buckwheat greens and will be mentioned in the upcoming discussion of wheatgrass, sunflower greens are seven-day-old greens grown from whole sunflower seeds on an inch of soil. For growing instructions, see *The Sprouting Book* by Ann Wigmore. Organically-grown sunflower greens are an excellent substitute for store-bought greens that have been commercially grown.

The juice of sunflower greens is best mixed with other vegetable juices as it tends to be rather bland and slimy. Sunflower green juice is rich in chlorophyll; vitamins A, B-1, B-2, C, niacin; the minerals calcium, magnesium, potassium, and proteins. It strengthens the gall bladder, liver, circulatory, and lymphatic systems, and the heart. Because it is high in calcium, it is soothing and cleansing to the digestive tract.

Selection

Choose greens that are fresh and with deep green leaves.

Yield

Four to six ounces juice per pound of sunflower greens.

Responsive Conditions

- Arthritis
- Asthma
- Bladder Disorders
- Cancer
- Circulatory Weakness
- Eye Disorders
- Heart Disease
- Kidney Disorders
- Liver Disorders
- Lung Disorders
- Skin Disorders
- Weight Loss

Sweet Pepper Juice

The juices of green and red peppers are pleasant tasting and mild compared to their spicy relatives, the hot green and red peppers. Taken as a beverage, hot pepper juice is quite disagreeable.

The difference between sweet green and sweet red peppers is age: the sweet red pepper is simply a ripe sweet green pepper. It has long been said that fruits and vegetables with shiny skins are high in potassium and silicon. This not an old wives' tale. Both green and red peppers are rich in these nutrients as well as vitamin C (the fully-ripe red pepper is rich in vitamin A, as well). This nutrient combination helps transfer the qualities of sweet pepper skins to us: that is, tightness and a healthy glow. Not simply skin beautifiers, both sweet red and sweet green peppers are wonderful flavor enhancers when used in green drinks and other vegetable juices.

Both varieties of sweet pepper juice are beneficial to the hair and nails as well as the skin. Sweet red pepper juice stimulates circulation and tones and cleanses the arteries and the heart muscle, as well.

Selection

Choose firm, shiny sweet peppers, preferably those that have not been waxed. Before juicing, wash gently with a mild castile soap.

Yield

Four to six ounces juice per pound of sweet peppers.

Responsive Conditions

- Arthritis
- Circulatory Weakness
- Eye Disorders
- Hair Loss
- Heart Disease
- High Blood Pressure
- Skin Disorders

Tomato Juice (Fresh)

Uncooked, fresh-squeezed tomato juice tastes and looks quite different from its salted, cooked, and canned counterpart. Cooked and uncooked tomato juice have opposite effects on the body. Canned tomatoes or tomato juice contains citric, malic, and oxalic acids. Made from cooked tomatoes, canned juice tends to acidify the blood and draw minerals from the tissues, teeth, and bones. Uncooked, vine-ripened tomatoes, or fresh-squeezed tomato juice, on the other hand, is slightly alkalizing. It adds to the stores of minerals—especially calcium—in the body.

Fresh tomato juice is also rich in vitamin C, and is highly cleansing to the liver. Fresh tomato juice stimulates circulation and the heart, and adds to the texture and flavor of fresh juices it is used in.

Hothouse tomatoes should not be used to make fresh tomato juice. These are the varieties that are available in the North during winter months. These types are picked green, shipped, and then gassed to make them turn a pink-red color.

Selection

Use only vine-ripened tomatoes for juicing, preferably from your garden, or from another local source during the summer growing season only.

Yield

Eight to ten ounces juice per pound of tomatoes.

Responsive Conditions

- Bladder Disorders
- Gall Bladder Disorders
- Gout
- Liver Disorders
- Kidney Disorders
- Skin Disorders
- Weight Loss

Turnip and Turnip Green Juice

Turnip greens stand out from all other vegetables in the amount of valuable calcium they contain. Ounce for ounce, turnip green juice actually contains more calcium than milk.

The turnip root contains calcium as well as potassium. Together, turnip root and green juices help neutralize overly acidic blood, and strengthen bones, hair, nails, and teeth. It is best to mix the juices of turnips and turnip greens with juices of alfalfa sprouts, dandelion greens, parsley, savoy cabbage, spinach, and sweet peppers. All these are high in magnesium. Magnesium helps the body to use calcium more effectively.

If turnip greens are not available where you shop, use store-bought collard or kale greens until it is warm enough to plant your own turnips. You can easily grow these plants in the spring and again in the late summer. They are very hardy plants. Plant them as soon as the earth is thawed, and harvest them early in the morning, right up to the time of the first snowfall.

Selection

Choose turnips that are firm and turnip greens that are deep green.

Yield

Four to six ounces juice per bunch of turnip greens. Four to six ounces of juice per pound of turnips.

Responsive Conditions

- Acne
- Anemia
- Arthritis
- Asthma
- Bladder Disorders
- Bronchitis
- Cancer
- Circulatory Disorders
- Diabetes

- Eye Disorders
- Heart Disease
- Infection
- Kidney Disorders
- Liver Disorders
- Lung Disorders
- Skin Disorders
- Weight Loss

Watercress Juice

Watercress is a delicate leafy green vegetable that contains more liquid than parsley, and has a slightly pungent taste. Watercress juice is a powerful cleanser, and a good source of vitamin C, calcium, and potassium. It is also rich in acid-forming minerals such as chorine, phosphorus, and sulfur, making it a first class intestinal cleanser and normalizer.

In addition, watercress juice is an excellent source of chlorophyll; it stimulates oxygen metabolism, circulatory functions, and the heart. Used for weight loss, watercress juice quickens metabolism and thus aids the conversion, of fat to energy. It is also useful in preventing menstrual discomfort.

Since watercress juice is strong in both effect and flavor, it is best used in combination with other juices. One ounce mixed with other vegetable juices is plenty.

Selection

Choose fresh, deep green colored watercress.

Yield

One to two ounces juice per bunch of watercress.

Responsive Conditions

- Anemia
- Bladder Disorders
- Circulatory Disorders
- Hair Loss
- Intestinal Disorders
- Kidney Disorders

- Liver Disorders
- Female Endocrine Imbalance
- Skin Disorders
- Thyroid Gland Regulation
- Weight Loss

Wheatgrass Juice

Wheatgrass is seven-inch-tall grass, grown from wheatberries on one inch of soil. Wheatgrass juice is perhaps the most nutritious and cleansing juice there is. Ann Wigmore has been responsible for the popularity of wheatgrass juice. In *The Wheatgrass Book*, she provides a detailed description of wheatgrass, its properties, uses, and remarkable regenerative and anti-aging abilities—as well as methods of growing and juicing wheatgrass. Let's look at a few of the more important points discussed in the book.

Wheatgrass juice contains many anti-aging properties. Among these are super oxide dismutase (S.O.D.); vitamins A,

B complex, C, and E; chlorophyll; a full spectrum of minerals and trace elements including calcium, iron, magnesium, and potassium; a number of special enzymes; and amino acids (proteins). But a more important, yet less understood, ingredient contained in wheatgrass is called the "grass juice factor." The grass juice factor is a property of wheatgrass that enables it to sustain life in herbivorous mammals indefinitely. No other single plant will keep mice, guinea pigs, cows, or sheep alive and well through generations. In other animal experiments, wheatgrass was able to return full potency in less than two months to male and female cows that had been unable to produce offspring.

Wheatgrass juice benefits the blood cells, bones, glands, hair, kidneys, liver, muscles, spleen, teeth, and other body parts. It can also be applied to the skin or scalp; implanted rectally to cleanse and heal the large intestine; or used to wash the eyes, gums, sinuses, and teeth.

Wheatgrass juice protects the lungs and blood from air and water pollution, cigarette smoke, toxins, and heavy metals. It is also a safe and extremely potent aid to weight loss. It works by suppressing appetite, and by stimulating metabolism and circulation.

Wheatgrass juice is an essential part of Ann Wigmore's Hippocrates Diet, and has been used for years by her guests. It is best mixed with other juices or taken alone in one- to three-ounce servings. For best results, sip fresh-squeezed wheatgrass juice on an empty or near-empty stomach, taking a couple of minutes to finish. If you are interested in knowing more about the uses of wheatgrass and its juice, refer to *The Wheatgrass Book* by Ann Wigmore.

Selection

Choose fresh, deep green colored wheatgrass.

Yield

Six to eight ounces juice per pound of wheatgrass, using a wheatgrass juicer.

Responsive Conditions

- Acne
- Aging (Premature)
- Anemia
- Arthritis
- Asthma
- Bladder Disorders
- Blood Pressure
  (High or Low)
- Bone Disorders
- Bronchitis
- Cancer
- Circulatory Weakness
- Colitis
- Constipation
- Diabetes
- Eye Disorders
- Fatigue
- Hay Fever
- Hair Loss
- Heart Disease
- Hypoglycemia
- Impotence
- Infection
- Kidney Disorders
- Liver Disorders
- Lung Disorders
- Nervous Disorders
- Skin Disorders
- Ulcers
- Weight Loss

5

The Cleansing Power of Fresh Fruit Juices: Apple to Watermelon

Packed with vitamins and purifying natural acidity, the fresh-squeezed juices of fruits have been dubbed the "body cleansers." Their natural counterparts are "the body restorers"—that is, the mineral-packed juices of fresh vegetables, sprouts, grasses, and greens. In the pages that follow, you'll learn about the benefits of a variety of fruit juices—from apple to watermelon. When combined in a long-term juice therapy program, the body cleansers and the body builders can work together to achieve and maintain health and well being.

For those who wish to read about a juice relative to a particular condition, the following chart provides information for referral. Conclusions represented by this information were arrived at after careful research, interviews with scores of health professionals including medical doctors and nutritionists, and with other recognized experts in the fields of preventive medicine, natural foods, and nutrition. The balance of this chapter provides an overview of each fruit listed in this chart. For further information, Appendix A correlates vitamins, minerals, bodily actions, and deficiency symptoms for fruits commonly used to make fresh juices.

This chart should not be used in place of qualified medical advice. Only a trained physician can diagnose and treat serious and degenerative illness.

Table 5.1   Fruit Juice Troubleshooting Chart

Condition	Recommended Fruit Juices
Acidosis	Papaya, Pineapple
Acne	Papaya, Strawberry
Aging (Premature)	Watermelon
Anemia	Cherry, Grape, Lemon, Lime, Orange, Prune
Arthritis	Apple, Cherry, Watermelon
Asthma	Cranberry
Bladder Disorders	Cranberry, Melon, Pear, Watermelon
Blood Disorders	Grape, Lemon, Lime, Orange, Papaya, Peach, Pineapple, Watermelon
Bruises	Grapefruit
Cancer	Grape
Colds	Grapefruit, Lemon, Lime, Orange, Pineapple
Constipation	Cherry, Grape, Lemon, Lime, Melon, Papaya, Peach, Pear, Prune Strawberry, Watermelon
Cough	Lemon, Lime
Cramps	Cherry
Diarrhea	Cranberry
Ear Disorders	Grapefruit, Lemon, Lime
Fever	Cranberry, Grape, Grapefruit, Lemon, Lime, Orange, Strawberry

Condition	Recommended Fruit Juices
Fluid Retention	Cranberry, Strawberry, Watermelon
Gall Stones	Cherry
Gout	Apple, Cherry, Grape, Lemon, Lime, Orange, Pineapple, Strawberry
Heart Disease	Orange, Papaya
Hemorrhoids	Grape
High Blood Pressure	Orange
Indigestion	Apple, Cherry, Cranberry, Grape, Grapefruit, Lemon, Lime, Orange, Papaya, Pineapple, Peach
Kidney Disorders	Apple, Cranberry, Grape, Melon, Papaya, Strawberry, Watermelon
Liver Disorders	Apple, Grapefruit, Grape, Lemon, Lime, Orange, Papaya, Pear
Mucous Membranes (including Catarrh Elimination)	Cherry, Grape, Grapefruit, Lemon, Lime, Orange
Pains	Strawberry, Watermelon
Pneumonia	Grapefruit, Lemon, Lime, Orange, Pineapple, Strawberry
Pregnancy	Grapefruit, Peach, Watermelon
Prostate Disorders	Cherry, Pear, Strawberry, Watermelon
Pyorrhea	Grapefruit, Lemon, Lime, Orange, Pineapple, Strawberry

Table 5.1   Fruit Juice Troubleshooting Chart, continued

Condition	Recommended Fruit Juices
Rheumatism	Apple, Cherry, Grape, Lemon, Lime, Orange, Strawberry
Sciatica	Pineapple
Scurvy	Grapefruit, Lemon, Lime, Orange
Skin Disorders	Cranberry, Grape, Grapefruit, Melon, Lemon, Lime, Orange, Watermelon
Sore Throat	Lemon, Lime
Thyroid Gland Regulation	Strawberry
Tumors	Papaya
Ulcers	Papaya
Urinary Tract Infection	Cranberry
Varicose Veins	Grapefruit
Weight Loss	Apple, Cherry, Cranberry, Grape, Grapefruit, Lemon, Lime, Orange, Papaya, Pineapple, Prune, Strawberry, Watermelon

FRUIT SUGAR VERSUS REFINED SUGAR

Fresh fruits contain both complex carbohydrates and simple sugars. Complex carbohydrates are more healthful than simple sugars because they are more slowly digested than simple sugars. Their energy is released more evenly over a longer period than the short bursts of the simple sugars. Although not as desirable as complex carbohydrates, the simple sugars found in fresh fruits come packaged with vitamins, minerals, and fiber. In this way, they differ from refined, white cane sugar. The main health concern with refined, white cane sugar is that it is used in high concentrations associated with many junk foods that are "empty calorie foods." That is, they supply virtually no minerals, vitamins, complex carbohydrates, or fiber. Their only benefit is their sweet taste. The unbalanced energy of the sugars in such junk foods causes obesity, tooth decay, overacidic blood due to fermentation of the sugars in the stomach, and malnutrition. The latter occurs when there is a loss of hunger for balanced, health-producing food after becoming addicted to a junk foods diet. By comparison, it is difficult to overeat sugar in fruits or over*drink* sugar in fruit juices. The sweetest fruits are far more nutritionally balanced than sugar-packed junk foods. In short, it is unlikely that a person could become obese from overconsumption of sugar on a natural foods diet containing plenty of fresh fruit juice.

FRUITS ARE SOLAR STOREHOUSES

Fresh fruits are carriers of great stores of solar energy. The presence of this energy in fresh fruits—as well as in all raw foods—is what determines the difference between, say, an orange and a chewable vitamin C tablet. While the most solar energy any food can provide is found in its uncooked state, the most solar energy available of any uncooked food is found in fresh fruits. This is because fruits ripen more slowly than almost any other foods, all the while soaking up and storing valuable energy from the sun.

While most of us know that vitamin C improves resistance to infection and calcium strengthens bones, many people do not understand the way that eating foods rich in solar energy affects the body. To observe this effect, picture the clear, tight skin, shiny hair, and bright eyes of many native mountain, island, and jungle peoples around the world. Most of these societies eat an abundance of fresh, locally grown fruits. Now, compare the image of these peoples with that of the toxic, burdened look on the faces and in the eyes of many Westerners who subsist on a diet of as much as 50 percent canned and refined foods. The difference is obvious.

THE CLEANSING POWER OF FRESH FRUIT JUICES

We call fruit juices cleansers for specific reasons. Whereas juices made from sprouts, greens, and vegetables are mild cleansers, fresh fruit juices are strong cleansers. Rich in vitamin C, pure liquids, and the acids that give them their tartness, fruits have the ability to scour away waste and harmful bacteria in the tissues of our bodies.

The three most prevalent acids found in fruits are citric acid, tartaric acid, and malic acid. Citric acid is found most abundantly in lemon juice, followed by the juice of the lime, grapefruit, orange, cranberry, strawberry, raspberry, pineapple, peach, and tomato.

Though the right amount of citric acid is a good thing, too much is a bad thing. Excess citric acid in the system can make the blood too acidic. Blood may also become too acidic due to high sugar, fat, or protein intake. This usually occurs in older people who no longer need to eat the same quantities of food they ate when they were younger, but continue to do so. When the blood has become too acidic, the body "borrows" the alkaline minerals calcium and magnesium from its skeletal system and teeth. Eventually, if this condition persists, the bones become so weak that they may break due to a minor fall. A diet full of fresh, whole foods will help combat this weakening of the bones.

How much citric acid is enough? The amount that's right for you will be determined, in the long run, by your age and level of activity. Activity helps to metabolize citric acid. This is because, like sugars, citric acid is metabolized more quickly and thoroughly with activity. Generally speaking, younger people metabolize citric acid better and easier than older people. So, unless you are an adult who is quite active physically, it might be a good idea to limit consumption of citrus fruits and juices to three or four six-ounce servings per week.

Another important fruit acid, tartaric acid, is found most abundantly in grapes and pineapples and, to a lesser extent, in many other commonly eaten fruits. Louis Pasteur, the French chemist, was the first to prove that this acid inhibits the growth of certain harmful molds and bacteria.

The fruit acid called malic acid is contained in apples, apricots, bananas, cherries, grapes, lemons, peaches, plums, prunes, and to a lesser degree in most other fruits. It is an excellent antiseptic. It cleanses the intestines, kidneys, liver, and stomach; and is a valuable aid in cleansing intestinal infection or distress. Malic acid also stimulates the appetite.

ENZYMES IN FRESH JUICES

Behind the powerful anti-bacterial action of the acids contained in fresh fruit juices are many potent enzymes. Pineapple and papaya enzymes, for example, have been used for decades to make enzyme supplements, due to their ability to digest protein and fats.

The enzymes in fresh fruit juices help flush the entire gastrointestinal system by digesting and neutralizing excess protein and fat found there. If consumed on a regular basis, fruit enzymes in fresh fruit juices can also enter the bloodstream and aid in cleansing the tissues, organs, and muscles of these same excesses. Fruit juices that are relatively high in calories, such as berry, grape, guava, mango, orange, papaya, persimmon, and pineapple juices, are higher in enzymes than juices made from apples, pears, or watermelon. However, all fresh fruit juices contain valuable enzymes that aid in digestion and internal cleansing.

FLUIDS IN FRESH JUICES

In addition to the host of nutrients mentioned here, fresh fruit juices supply purified liquids to the body. Unlike commercially sold distilled water that is ionized, then heated, then cooled, the water from a fruit tree or vine is filtered through the roots and branches and energized by the entire plant in its growth cycle.

The action of the liquids contained in fresh fruit juice is similar to the action of glacial waters that flow through the Hunza region of Pakistan. People who drink the water there live extraordinarily long and vigorous lives—many to ages of 100 to 120 years. Like mineral water that has been distilled naturally, the fluids in fresh fruit juices add minerals to the body, reduce acidity, and thus contribute to healthy bones and teeth.

In varying degrees, all fruit juices have cleansing abilities. I have found the juices of apple, grape, lemon, orange, and pineapple to be especially helpful in problems of hyperacidity, fever, colds, sore throat, internal or external infection, obesity, and low energy due to bodily toxicity. And as a preventive health measure for children, fresh fruit juices can't be beat. It's natural for kids to love them and they're good for them in moderate amounts—that is, four 6-ounce servings per week.

Now that we know that fresh fruit juices can play a role in helping us to live cleaner, healthier, and longer lives, what are we waiting for? Let's take a look at the beneficial characteristics of a variety of fresh fruit juices we can make at home.

Apple Juice

There are many varieties of apples from which to choose. Cortland, Golden Delicious, Granny Smith, McIntosh, Pippin, and others are available at most markets across the country. All of these are fine for juicing. Harder, crisper apples are best for juicing. Mushy or grainy apples tend to become soupy when juiced. Waxed apples should be peeled and washed before juicing. Organically grown or unwaxed apples need only to be washed and juiced with the seeds for maximum taste and nutrition.

Fresh apple juice made from unpeeled apples is rich in vitamins and minerals. In it are substantial amounts of vitamins A, B-1, B-2, B-6, C, biotin, folic acid, pantothenic acid, and a host of minerals, among them, chlorine, copper, iron, magnesium, manganese, phosphorus, potassium, silicon, sodium, and sulfur. Due to its high mineral content, fresh apple juice is especially good for the health of the skin, hair, and fingernails.

It is important to note that the juice of peeled apples will yield half as much vitamin A as the juice of unpeeled apples. This is because a high percentage of the vitamin A in apples is concentrated in their skins. Therefore, the apple juice with the highest vitamin A content will be the apple juice from unpeeled, organically grown apples that are juiced with their skins on.

The vitamin C content of fresh juice from both peeled and unpeeled apples helps prevent colds, flu, and intestinal infections. It helps activate the body's elaborate defense system against bacterial toxins. The substantial amount of fruit pectin contained in fresh apple juice is responsible for its often thick texture and cloudiness. Pectin forms a gel in our intestines, absorbs and dissolves toxins, and stimulates peristaltic activity, the wavelike motion of the large intestine that helps it move food through the digestive tract. This normalizes elimination due to either constipation or diarrhea. Apple juice and apple cider owe their reputations as bowel regulators to the pectin and malic acid contained in them.

Fresh apple juice blends well with other juices. For instance, fresh apple juice mixed with an equal amount of fresh carrot juice and three tablespoons of fresh beet juice makes a sweet, blood-building drink.

Selection

Choose apples that are not waxed or sprayed, if possible, to avoid having to peel them. Often the smaller apples sold in bags by the pound are unwaxed. If your produce manager confirms they have not been grown with harmful pesticides, they will be excellent for juicing. Also look for firm apples, as mealy apples will not yield much juice.

Yield

Six to eight ounces juice per pound of apples.

Responsive Conditions

- Arthritis
- Constipation
- Gout
- Indigestion

- Kidney Disorders
- Liver Disorders
- Rheumatism
- Weight Loss

Cherry Juice

Fresh cherry juice, though more time-consuming to make than apple juice, is well worth the effort. By using a cherry pitter and running pitted cherries through a juicer, you can make one of the best-tasting and most healthful fresh juices there is. However, since cherry juice is quite rich, it is best to mix it with equal parts of apple juice, water, or another fresh fruit juice.

Fresh cherry juice is especially rich in vitamins A and C. It also contains vitamins B-1, B-2, folic acid, and niacin. Minerals in cherry juice include calcium, cobalt, florine, iron, magnesium phosphorus, and potassium. Fresh cherry juice is a powerful alkalizer and therefore reduces the acidity of the blood. For this reason, it is especially effective in cases of gout and arthritis. Cherry juice is also effective in normalizing prostatic disorders.

Selection

Choose deep, dark colored cherries that are firm to the touch yet soft enough to be ripe. Pick through and discard any mushy fruit.

Yield

Six to eight ounces juice per pound of pitted cherries.

Responsive Conditions

- Anemia
- Arthritis
- Constipation
- Cramps
- Gall Stones
- Gout

- Indigestion
- Mucous Membranes (including Catarrh Elimination)
- Rheumatism
- Prostate Disorders
- Weight Loss

Cranberry Juice

Most cranberries marketed in the United States are grown in the Northeast. Cranberries grow in bogs, which are flooded in cold weather. During the fall and early winter, fresh cranberries are available at most supermarkets throughout the country. Since cranberry juice is sour-tasting and acidic, it is best to mix small amounts of it with apple or other fresh fruit juices.

Fresh cranberry juice is rich in vitamins A, C, B complex, and folic acid. It contains minerals, including calcium, iron, phosphorus, potassium, sodium, and sulfur. For years, hospital staffs have served their patients cranberry juice because it is a natural diuretic and urinary tract cleanser. Unfortunately, the cranberry juice that hospitals use is often processed and bottled. It contains corn syrup and refined sugar which makes it a less pure, sugar-laden drink—not pure juice. In processing, its enzymes are destroyed. By comparison, fresh-pressed cranberry juice contains very little sugar and is full of live enzymes.

Cranberry juice contains substances called vasodilators that open blood vessels. When blood vesels in the bronchial tubes are dilated, breathing is easier. For this reason, cranberry juice can help provide temporary relief of lung congestion.

Selection

Choose cranberries that are deep-colored and firm.

Yield

Four to six ounces juice per pound of cranberries.

Responsive Conditions

- Asthma
- Bladder Disorders
- Diarrhea
- Fever
- Fluid Retention
- Indigestion

- Kidney Disorders
- Lung Disorders
- Skin Disorders
- Urinary Tract Infection
- Weight Loss

Grape Juice

Few foods are more tempting to the eyes and palate than a well-formed cluster of ripe, luscious grapes. Freshly juiced grapes are both sweet and nourishing. Almost any variety of grape is good for juicing, though some Concord varieties can be sour. Even these, however, taste great mixed with other juices.

After washing, grapes can be juiced—seeds and all. If the taste is too sweet, merely dilute the juice with an equal amount of spring water.

Fresh grape juice contains good supplies of vitamins A, B-1, B-2, C, and niacin. It provides an abundance of minerals, including calcium, chlorine, copper, fluorine, iron, magnesium, manganese, phosphorus, potassium, silicon, and sulfur. It is an excellent source of tartaric acid, and energy-producing natural sugars in unconcentrated form.

Fresh-squeezed grape juice is an excellent stimulator of the metabolism. A higher metabolism is desirable because it helps burn excess food and waste more rapidly than a low metabolism. While fresh-squeezed grape juice may help you lose weight by increasing your metabolism, its abundance of minerals helps cleanse and build the blood, and stimulates the liver to increase its cleansing activity.

Selection

Choose grapes that are fresh and firm to the touch. Deep-colored red and purple grapes are more flavorful, while green grapes that have turned slightly yellow due to ripening taste best.

Yield

Eight ounces juice per pound of grapes.

Responsive Conditions

- Anemia
- Blood Disorders
- Cancer
- Constipation
- Fever
- Gout
- Hemorrhoids
- Indigestion
- Kidney Disorders
- Liver Disorders
- Mucous Membranes (including Catarrh Elimination)
- Rheumatism
- Skin Disorders
- Weight Loss

Grapefruit Juice

The best grapefruits in America are grown in Florida and Texas. The pink and red varieties are more sweet and generally less acidic than white grapefruits. The best way to juice grapefruits, oranges, or lemons is the following: peel them, quarter them, discard the seeds, leave some white on the fruit, and run the wedges through a high-speed juicer. Juice made this way will be slightly creamy and far more rich in nutrients than juice that has simply been squeezed in a manual citrus juice squeezer.

Grapefruit juice is rich in vitamin C, and in the minerals calcium, phosphorus, and potassium. It contains lesser amounts of vitamins B complex, E, K, biotin, inositol, and various minerals.

The bioflavonoids in grapefruits are concentrated in the white pulp surrounding the fruit. Bioflavonoids help the body to retain and use vitamin C. Together, these two nutrients improve the permeability and strength of capillary walls. This is why citrus juice made as described here helps heal bruises more quickly than if they were not treated with citrus juice.

Pregnant women often crave grapefruit. This is probably because the bioflavonoids and vitamin C in them give strength to capillary walls that are taxed by the fluid retention and swelling that are common during pregnancy.

Though not last in importance by any means, common colds benefit greatly from a diet rich in citrus juices. Unfortunately, while convenient, pasteurized, frozen, and concentrated citrus juices do not produce the same health benefits as fresh-squeezed citrus juices. Fresh grapefruit juice, for example, will produce a light sweat and relieve a sore throat. Reconstituted frozen grapefruit juice may simply supply liquids to the system—an important consideration for the cold sufferer, but probably not the one that led him or her to purchase the grapefruit juice as a cold tonic.

Though grapefruit juice is a beneficial drink, it is most effective when taken in moderation. As you will recall from the discussion earlier in this chapter, citrus juices taken in excess can leech calcium from the system, softening bones and teeth. If you drink more than three to four 6-ounce glasses per week, make sure to get extra exercise to burn excess acid. Ultimately, the amount you choose should be tailored to your age and normal activity level. Younger, more active people will have higher metabolisms able to manage more citric acid. Older, less active people will have lower metabolisms and should therefore use less citrus juice.

Selection

Choose heavy grapefruits with thin skins as these tend to have more juice and flavor.

Yield

Six to eight ounces juice per pound of grapefruit.

Responsive Conditions

- Bruises
- Colds
- Ear Disorders
- Fever
- Indigestion
- Mucous Membranes (including Catarrh Elimination)

- Pregnancy
- Pyorrhea
- Scurvy
- Skin Disorders
- Varicose Veins
- Weight Loss

Lemon Juice

Lemon juice is perhaps the most valuable and versatile fruit juice. However, since its high citric acid and vitamin C content makes it such a strong cleanser, it is best to mix lemon juice with water and drink it in moderation. The juice of half a lemon combined with eight ounces of water is a good ratio. Add one-half teaspoonful of raw honey if you prefer, to lightly sweeten the drink. Lemon juice used every two or three days in this way is a great balancer. Try it before breakfast. It will act as a mild and completely safe cleanser of the small intestine and stomach when drunk before food is eaten.

In *Health Guide For Survival,* author Salem Kirban writes about biochemist Carey Reams and his theory of illness and health. Reams' suggested nutritional program involves, among other things, the use of lemon juice. Almost every food, with the exception of lemons, writes Kirban, produces cations (pronounced cat-eye-uns) in the blood and body. Cations are acidic substances with a positive ionic charge. Lemons, and our own digestive juices, on the other hand, are the only substances that produce anions (pronounced an-eye-uns), or alkaline substances with a negative ionic charge.

According to Reams' theory, we don't survive on the food we eat, but rather on the energy in the food we eat—energy created by the interchange between cations aned anions during digestion. Illness is brought about, Reams contends, when the body has fewer anions available to get energy from more plentiful cations in foods. Lemon juice's anionic properties restore the internal balance between cations and anions, and assist the liver in manufacturing many different enzymes that help digest cationic molecules in our food. The use of lemon juice, Reams concludes, increases energy levels and brings about metabolic balance.

Lemon juice has many other practical uses, as well. To relieve a sore throat, for example, squeeze or spray undiluted lemon juice directly into the throat every two hours. Its anti-bacterial action will soothe the throat in a few hours. Before you feel a cold coming on, drink several glasses of lemon water throughout the day. To use as a skin astringent, add lemon juice to water and apply after washing the skin with a mild soap. Lemon juice can also be used effectively as an antioxidant. Mixed with other juices, or in fruit salads, it not only prevents discoloration, but acts as a preservative, as well.

Selection

Choose firm lemons with thin skins, as these have the most juice and flavor.

Yield

Four to five ounces juice per pound of lemons.

Responsive Conditions

- Anemia
- Blood Disorders
- Colds
- Constipation
- Cough
- Ear Disorders
- Liver Disorders
- Mucous Membranes (including Catarrh Elimination)
- Pneumonia
- Pyorrhea
- Rheumatism

- Fever
- Gout
- Indigestion
- Infection

- Scurvy
- Skin Disorders
- Sore Throat
- Weight Loss

Lime Juice

Lime juice is similar to lemon juice in both effect and nutrition, though it is not as acidic and, therefore, is not as powerful a cleanser. Lime juice can be used as a substitute for lemon juice when desired. As with lemon juice, its strength can be controlled by mixing it with other juices or water before drinking.

Selection

Choose firm, heavy limes with thin skins, as these have the most juice and flavor.

Yield

Four to five ounces juice per pound of limes.

Responsive Conditions

- Anemia
- Blood Disorders
- Colds
- Constipation
- Cough
- Ear Disorders
- Fever
- Gout
- Indigestion
- Infection

- Liver Disorders
- Mucous Membranes (including Catarrh Elimination)
- Pneumonia
- Pyorrhea
- Rheumatism
- Scurvy
- Skin Disorders
- Sore Throat
- Weight Loss

Melon Juice

Melons—including canary, cantaloupe, casba, crenshaw, honeydew, and musk—produce great-tasting, energy-producing juices. Melon juices are summertime favorites with our family. Most melons have similar nutritional content. Cantaloupes and muskmelons are especially rich in vitamins A, B complex, and C. This makes them good skin and nerve food. All melons contain a variety of vitamins, minerals, enzymes, and plenty of natural, unconcentrated sugars. They are cooling and have a tonic effect on digestion.

Selection

Choose firm melons that have a sweet smell and a soft spot opposite the stem end. Heavy melons have more water content and therefore make better juice.

Yield

Six to eight ounces juice per pound of melon.

Responsive Conditions

- Bladder Disorders
- Constipation
- Kidney Disorders
- Skin Disorders

Orange Juice

Orange juice is America's favorite. Unfortunately, most commercially bottled and frozen orange juices are pasteurized. Pasteurization kills enzymes. Some commercially made juices contain added concentrated sugar. As we learned at the beginning of this chapter, these types of orange juice are, therefore, not recommended. Fresh-squeezed orange juice or peeled oranges juiced in a high-speed juicer are superior in taste and nutrition.

Fresh orange juice is rich in vitamins A and C, and contains lesser amounts of vitamins B-1, B-2, B-6, E, K, biotin, folic acid, inositol, niacin, bioflavonoids, and eleven amino acids. Oranges are supplied with an abundance of minerals, including calcium, chlorine, copper, fluorine, iron, manganese, magnesium, phosphorus, potassium, silicon, and zinc.

Like grapefruit and lemon juices, orange juice cleanses and tones the gastrointestinal tract. It also improves permeability and strength of capillary walls. Both the heart and lungs benefit from regular consumption of fresh orange juice. Overly acidic blood is alkalized by drinking orange juice on a regular basis in moderate amounts; that is, three to four 6-ounce glasses per week.

Selection

Choose firm, heavy juicing oranges with thin skins.

Yield

Six to eight ounces juice per pound of oranges.

Responsive Conditions

· Anemia	· Liver Disorders
· Blood Disorders	· Lung Disorders
· Colds	· Pneumonia
· Fever	· Pyorrhea
· Gout	· Rheumatism
· Heart Disease	· Scurvy
· High Blood Pressure	· Skin Disorders
· Indigestion	· Weight Loss

Papaya Juice

Most papayas sold in American supermarkets are shipped from Hawaii, where they are grown. Other producers of the papaya are the states of California, Florida, and Texas. Imported papayas are shipped to U.S. markets from the Caribbean, Central America, and Mexico.

The outer skin of a papaya turns yellow or orange when it is ripe, and the flesh becomes sweet and soft. To prepare them for juicing, cut in half, scoop out the seeds and discard, and then scoop out the flesh, throwing the skins away. Then run the flesh thrugh the juicer. Using a blender, you can also freeze and then blend the papaya spears with other fresh juices to make smoothies. (Smoothie recipes are found in Chapter 7.) To make plain papaya juice in a blender, simply blend two to four ounces of water with the flesh of one medium-sized papaya.

Papaya juice is rich in vitamins A and C, and contains small amounts of the minerals calcium, chlorine, iron, phosphorus, potassium, silicon, and sodium. Its nutritional highlight is its enzymes, specifically papain, a protein digestant. It is also endowed with an abundance of energy-boosting natural sugars when ripe. Papaya juice strengthens the body's blood coagulating ability. It is a fine laxative, appetite stimulant, and cleanser of the kidneys, liver, and intestines.

Selection

Choose papayas that have turned a deep gold, orange, or yellow. This signals that they are ripe. They should give a little when squeezed, yet not be mushy.

Yield

One to three ounces juice per pound of papaya. Both juicers and blenders may be used to make papaya juice.

Responsive Conditions

- Acidosis
- Acne
- Blood Disorders
- Constipation
- Heart Disease
- Indigestion

- Kidney Disorders
- Liver Disorders
- Tumors
- Ulcers
- Weight Loss

Peach Juice

Fresh peaches are among our family's favorite fruits. They may be eaten whole or juiced. Though fresh peach juice is somewhat thick, it can be diluted with water or mixed with apple or grape juice to thin it.

To prepare for juicing, wash peaches well, cut in quarters, and remove their pits. Then, run through the juicer.

Fresh peach juice is rich in vitamin A. It also contains vitamins B-1, B-2, C, niacin; and minerals including calcium, iron, phosphorus, potassium, and sodium. Peach juice cleanses the intestines and stimulates peristaltic activity of the lower bowel. Peach juice has been used successfully by pregnant women to prevent morning sickness and other prenatal difficulties.

Selection

Choose deep colored peaches that are firm but give a little when squeezed. If selecting fruit at your market, avoid overly green peaches. Even though they will soften after several days, green peaches will not be as sweet as peaches that are deep yellow or orange when displayed at your market. Of course, the sweetest and most nutritious peaches are tree ripened and deep colored.

Yield

One to three ounces juice per pound of peaches. Peaches may be used in place of papayas for blender drinks and smoothies. (These drinks are detailed in Chapter 7.)

Responsive Conditions

- Blood Disorders
- Constipation

- Indigestion
- Pregnancy

Pear Juice

Pear juice is thick and very sweet. Bosc, Anjou, or Bartlett pears all make fine juice. Pear juice can be diluted with water and lemon juice or apple juice if desired.

To juice pears, wash and remove hard stems, cut, and run through the juicer either by themselves or with other fruits and vegetables.

Pear juice contains vitamins A, B-1, B-2, C, folic acid, and niacin. It is also rich in phosphorus and potassium, and supplies lesser amounts of calcium, chlorine, iron, magnesium, sodium, and sulfur. Pear juice has mild diuretic and laxative effects.

Selection

Choose firm, deep colored green, gold, or red pears. Let them sit for a few days, if needed, until they give a little when squeezed. Do not juice mushy pears, as they will produce little juice.

Yield

Four to six ounces juice per pound of pears.

Responsive Conditions

- Bladder Disorders
- Constipation

- Liver Disorders
- Prostate Disorders

Pineapple Juice

Fresh-squeezed pineapple juice is sweet, delicious, and thirst-quenching. Choose pineapples that have golden-colored skin.

Smell them. If they smell strong and sweet, they are ripe.

To prepare for juicing, remove top and bottom of fruit and peel skin from sides. Juice the meat.

Fresh pineapple juice is rich in vitamin C, and the minerals chlorine and potassium. It contains an abundance of other vitamins and minerals, as well as the enzyme bromelin. Bromelin has many uses in the body, among them, its buffering ability. Bromelin helps the body to balance and neutralize fluids that are either too alkaline or too acidic. Bromelin also stimulates hormonal secretions in the pancreas. For this reason, pineapple is used in the commercial production of certain hormones. Pineapple juice also works effectively to soothe sore throats because of its high content of vitamin C, enzymes, and fruit acids.

Selection

Choose pineapples that have golden-colored skin, smell strong and sweet, and give a little when pressed.

Yield

Four to six ounces juice per pound of pineapple.

Responsive Conditions

- Acidosis
- Blood Disorders
- Colds
- Gout
- Indigestion
- Pneumonia
- Pyorrhea
- Sciatica
- Weight Loss

Prune Juice

Prunes are a variety of dried plums. To juice them, you will need to use a blender and a strainer. Soak fifteen pitted prunes in a quart of hot water overnight. Blend the prunes with the water in which they were soaked. Strain the juice and discard the pulp, if you wish. You may dilute the juice with spring water or drink undiluted.

Prune juice is a good source of vitamin A and the minerals copper and iron. The benzoic and quinic acids in prune juice make it an excellent laxative.

Selection

Choose large, sweet pitted prunes.

Yield

Sixteen to twenty-four ounces juice per each group of fifteen dried prunes, soaked overnight, and blended with water, depending on desired consistency.

Responsive Conditions

- Anemia
- Constipation
- Weight Loss

Strawberry Juice

Fresh spring strawberries make excellent juice. Since it is strong and somewhat thick, strawberry juice may be mixed with apple juice, citrus juice, or water. To prepare fresh strawberries for juicing, wash them thoroughly and remove green tops. Then, juice whole.

Strawberry juice is rich in vitamin C, and the minerals calcium, phosphorus, and potassium. It is also one of the few fruit juices that contains natural painkillers. These substances, called organic salyicilates, are a basic ingredient of painkillers such as aspirin. Spring's strawberry juice is highly cleansing to the blood, tissues, and muscles—in short, Nature's answer to a long winter indoors. It can also be used effectively as a mild diuretic.

Selection

It is best to use locally grown strawberries in season. This is because many berries grown in foreign countries or shipped across the country tend not to be as sweet and flavorful, or as juicy. In addition, there are many objectionable chemicals used to grow commercial strawberries that are shipped across the country or imported from other countries. For more information, refer to the Consumer Alerts on pesticides in Chapter 7.

Yield

Four to five ounces juice per pound of strawberries.

Responsive Conditions

· Acne	· Pains
· Constipation	· Pneumonia
· Fluid Retention	· Pyorrhea
· Fever	· Rheumatism
· Gout	· Thyroid Disorders
· Kidney Disorders	· Weight Loss

Watermelon Juice

Watermelon juice is an all-time favorite of ours. During the summer, we juice the entire fruit—rind, seeds, and all. It makes a sweet, greenish-brown-colored juice.

Whole watermelon juice is rich in vitamin A and the mineral potassium. It contains lesser amounts of many other vitamins, minerals, and chlorophyll. Those who prefer less sugar in their juices will be interested to know that the juice of the whole watermelon is less sweet than the juice of the red meat alone. By juicing the rind, you will increase its mineral and chlorophyll content.

Watermelon juice is a top-notch kidney and bladder cleanser. Its diuretic action helps to eliminate excess fluids from the body. Watermelon juice is also endowed with plenty of enzymes. It is a natural appetite stimulant. Juiced whole, watermelon can be drunk throughout the day—between meals or before bedtime. Keep watermelon in the refrigerator year-round to enjoy its healthful juice.

Selection

Choose well-shaped watermelons with smooth, hard skin.

Yield

Six to eight ounces juice per pound of watermelon.

Responsive Conditions

- Aging (Premature)
- Arthritis
- Bladder Disorders
- Blood Disorders
- Constipation
- Fluid Retention
- Kidney Disorders
- Pregnancy
- Prostate Disorders
- Skin Disorders
- Weight Loss

6
Juice Fasting

To fast is to go without any food or certain types of food for a period of time. Fasting is perhaps the quickest method of eliminating toxins from the body, while also allowing the digestive system to rest and repair itself. However, while some fasts are beneficial, others are harmful. Often-recommended water fasts, for example, or extended fasting of any kind can be dangerous.

Juice fasting offers the satisfaction of fasting and cleansing the body in one of the quickest ways possible. Best of all, it accomplishes its task with complete safety. Juice fasting is drinking only fresh fruit or vegetable juice for a one to three day period. In this chapter, we will discuss the benefits of these brief juice fasts and outline a safe and effective cleansing/fasting program.

THE BENEFITS OF FASTING

Why is it that when we become ill, we often lose our appetites? Why do you suppose that sick pets refuse to eat? It is because, in times of physical crisis, the body attempts to correct and balance that physical crisis. A short fast brought on by nausea leaves us feeling better, with more energy, and a healthy appetite.

Water fasting has been recommended by many health educators in Europe and America for over a century. The idea of fasting in Western culture began with Hippocrates and his mono (single food) diets. He served his patients whole-grain barley that was ground and cooked into meal (gruel) along with water or diluted wine. The idea was that by simplifying food and liquid intake, the body's natural self-healing, cleansing, and regenerating abilities would speed recovery. But Hippocrates was not the only historic figure to recommend fasting. The Bible contains many references to fasting. Jesus fasted with his disciples on many occasions, not only to heal disease, but for spiritual uplifting—to overcome the desires of the flesh. Centuries before Jesus, Hindus and Buddhists were practicing fasting for similar reasons.

After three thousand years, however, the methods of fasting introduced by Hippocrates have been abandoned. Absent from the teachings of modern preventive medicine is the common-sense information that fasting cleanses the body through eliminative channels. Modern preventive medicine omits fasting and instead focuses its emphasis on feeding the body; on vitamins, exercise, and sleep habits. Yet, in order to remain healthy, the body's eliminative organs must function efficiently, as well. While poor elimination may not be the sole cause of disease, it should not be discounted as a contributing factor.

Brief juice fasts that help the eliminative process are an ideal preventive health measure. During a juice fast, the body is stimulated to greater metabolic and eliminative activity. Pounds are shed, the skin tightens and clears, hair shines, eyes brighten, the intestines and other digestive organs rest and purge themselves, and less sleep is required.

Many who perform this fast report experiencing a physical "high." Unlike the post-Thanksgiving holiday laziness and sleepiness many report as a result of overeating, most juice-fasters attest to feeling stronger and more energetic, both physically and mentally. Many people prefer to eat lightly when traveling or when focusing attention for prolonged periods of mental work. Brief juice fasts such as those described in this chapter can be used by healthy adults to increase energy levels and mental clarity.

Juice fasting can also boost the faster's confidence through the experience of discipline and self-control required to perform the fast. Once you prove to yourself that you can fast for three days, you may feel more in control of your diet as well as other aspects of your life. Through fasting, you learn by doing that you control your body and your appetite—not the opposite.

But, psychological benefits aside, it is wise to keep in perspective the main purpose of juice fasting: to keep the body healthy. You can consider the mental and emotional gains derived from fasting as "spiritual dividends."

If you are at all apprehensive about juice fasting, you are probably not ready for it. You may never be. But don't lose heart. You can cleanse and repair your body more slowly, but similarly, by eating a "whole foods diet," rich in whole grains, beans, fresh vegetables, fruits, and other foods that have not been processed, de-natured, or altered; and by drinking plenty of fresh juices. In fact, for many folks, especially those with health problems and the elderly, it is probably best to add whole foods and fresh juices to the regular diet before attempting a fast.

PHYSICAL CHANGES DURING THE FAST

If you follow the recommendations set forth in this chapter closely, physical discomfort during juice fasts will be minimal. It is possible that you may experience minor irritations such as runny nose, sore muscles, temporary fatigue, loss of appetite, and so on. However, these symptoms will pass; and when they do, you will feel better both physically and mentally. If, for some reason, a symptom arising during the fast persists for several days, merely discontinue the fast.

PERFORMING THE FAST

Try not to push yourself too hard while fasting. Keep the one to three days as free as possible of appointments or errands. Instead, relax, read, do light exercise, work in the yard, or go to the beach. If you feel the urge to sleep, do so. As long as you drink the recommended two-to-three quarts of liquid each day, extra sleep will do your body good. Normally, you will require less sleep during fasting, as less sleep is required to balance body functions.

If you are so inclined, take a simple warm-water enema every morning of the fast. An enema will speed the removal of waste from the large intestine.

In place of regular meals, drink one or two 8-ounce glasses of fresh vegetable or fruit juice. These can be drunk "as-is" or diluted with spring water. If you become thirsty between meals of fresh juice, drink another glass of juice, or lemon water that has been sweetened lightly with raw honey or pure maple syrup. Drink enough glasses of juice and lemon water equal to a total of two to three quarts of liquid each day.

BREAKING THE FAST

After the fast, let your body adjust to solid foods at first. There is a tendency for fasters to wake up on the morning after the fast and to eat everything in sight! It is much better to break the fast with a breakfast (or dinner if you are breaking your fast at night) of simple foods such as fresh fruits or steamed vegetables. By the time you are hungry for a second meal, you can resume normal light eating. Keep in mind, however, that the stomach shrinks considerably during fasting. Smaller portions of food eaten more often will prevent the uncomfortable feeling of overeating that may occur when breaking a fast.

FASTING DO'S AND DONT'S

You may have to adjust the juice fast to your own needs and desires. This section will give you some guidelines for getting the most from a juice fast. For example, the recommendation to drink two to three quarts of liquid per day is vital to the fasting process and if ignored could cause dehydration. The way you break the fast is also important: take small, simple meals more often until the stomach expands to its pre-fast condition.

Fast for one day, two days, or a full three days. If halfway through the first day you feel that it will be too stressful to continue fasting, simply break the fast as instructed. If the fasting process is going to be one long punishment for you, it's better to change it to suit your needs, or to abandon it altogether.

To some degree, during any type of fast, the blood pools in the abdominal region of your body. There is nothing bad about having more blood in this area, but it does mean that there is less blood in the head. This could cause dizziness if you attempt too many quick starts. So exercise care in your activities.

Many people experience surges of energy during one or all of the days. They have an urge to set new records for the number of miles they can walk or hours they can work. Try not to overdo it. Instead, be moderate and channel your energy into the internal housecleaning that is taking place. Some mild exercise will be beneficial. But avoid hours of walking or overly-strenuous work.

Also, try to stay close to home. Traveling during fasting is not advised, especially driving long distances. In certain ways the mind and reflexes may not be as sharp during your initial fast. Caution should be your guide. If possible, spend lots of time outdoors in the sun, tinkering in your garden, and so on. Sunlight will stimulate various body-cleansing processes. For this reason, I recommend juice fasting in sunny weather—preferably in spring and summer. Once you have performed your first juice fast successfully, you can tailor your next fast to your own special needs.

SUMMARY

The following summary of a typical day on a juice fast may serve as a handy reference guide. Use this guide during your fast:

· Begin each day of the fast with a simple warm water enema, if you are so inclined.

· Each morning drink one or two glasses of fresh vegetable or fruit juice.

- Between breakfast and lunch you may drink another glass of juice or lemon water if desired. Drink one to two glasses of vegetable or green juice for lunch, and have the same for dinner. You may substitute fruit juice if desired.

- Get plenty of rest and relaxation. Do some light stretching and walking. Spend lots of time out of doors. And don't force yourself to follow a schedule or meet deadlines.

- Break the fast after either a few hours; or one, two, or three days with a simple meal of fresh fruit or steamed vegetables.

If these recommendations are followed, your first fast should be a happy and worthwhile adventure in self-education, and self-help. It will enable you to take a giant step forward in safeguarding your future health and happiness.

7
Fresh Juice Recipes

It's easy to prepare fresh juices. All you need are high-quality raw materials and the appropriate juicer.

It's important to choose the freshest and ripest produce available. Rubbery vegetables, wilted greens and grasses, and over- or under-ripe fruits will produce juices that are neither tasty nor healthful.

Likewise, your choice of juicer is important. To prepare the recipes in this chapter, you will need two models: a high-speed juicer and a wheatgrass juicer. In addition, a blender may be used in place of a high-speed juicer to prepare the smoothies in this chapter.

Use a high-speed juicer to prepare the following recipes for fresh fruit and vegetable juices and a wheatgrass juicer to prepare the green drinks and wheatgrass juices. For help in selecting the proper type of juicer, refer to Chapter 3.

The next step is to remove all traces of pesticide, fertilizer, soil, and wax from your juicing materials. To learn more about pesticides and what you can do about them, refer to the following Consumer Alert boxes. Carrots, beets, and other root vegetables—whether organically or inorganically grown—should be scrubbed thoroughly with mild castile or coconut-based soap and water. Carefully rinse or soak greens, grasses, and sprouts in cold water. For maximum potency, choose organically-grown produce. Peel waxed apples and cucumbers.

Consumer Alert: Pesticides

The abundance, variety, and freshness of the fruits and vegetables commonly found on supermarket shelves is made possible, in part, by the ongoing use of chemical fertilizers, pesticides, and herbicides. While safe forms of these crop boosters are now available, the majority of the farming industry continues to use a variety of fertilizers, pesticides, coolants, and gasses that have been proven to be unsafe in laboratory experiments on animals. And despite governmental efforts to curb or control their use, residues of these chemicals remain in and on our food.

While the general public is unaware of the extent of pesticide and herbicide contamination, the United States Food and Drug Administration (FDA) has revealed that it is a widespread problem. A February 1987 report by the U.S. Environmental Protection Agency (EPA), "Unfinished Business," considered the presence of pesticides in food to be one of this nation's most serious health and environmental problems.

Between 1982 and 1985, the FDA's laboratories detected pesticide residues in 48 percent of the most frequently consumed fresh fruits and vegetables. And since the FDA can routinely detect only about half of the pesticides in random samples of less than one percent of our food, there is reason to believe the problem is understated.

It is only by confronting the FDA and demanding changes—as with the banning of Alar, the pesticide proven to cause cancer in children—that the public will influence governmental policy toward this problem.

For more information on pesticides in fresh food, you may want to consult the Natural Resources Defense Council's 1988 publication, *Pesticide Alert*, by Lawrie Mott and Karen Snyder (Sierra Club Books, San Francisco). The book lists twenty-six common varieties of fresh fruits and vegetables, the pesticides most frequently found on and inside each food, the health effects associated with those pesticides, and what you can do about removing them.

Consumer Alert: Reducing Exposure

Where you buy your produce, what you buy, and how you prepare it can reduce exposure to pesticides. Here are some tips:

- Buy organically grown produce. Alternative methods to pest and weed control have been available to commercial farmers for years, and are gaining in popularity. Certified organically grown foods should contain almost no pesticides.
- Wash all produce. This will remove some, but not all, of the pesticides. A mild solution of pure castile soap available at natural foods stores, water, and a vegetable scrub brush will remove additional surface pesticide residues.
- Peel produce and remove the outer leaves when appropriate. In many cases, the loss of nutrients found close to the skin or in the outer leaves outweighs the exposure to pesticides and waxes. Peeling fruits such as apples, pears, avocadoes, peaches, and pineapples, or vegetables such as bell peppers, parsnips, turnips, cucumber, and tomatoes, will remove all surface pesticides and waxes used to preserve them. Removing outer leaves of lettuces, cabbages, and other vegetables also helps.
- Buy domestically grown produce, and buy it in season. Many of the imported foods tested by the government have far greater concentrations of pesticide residues. Foreign governments tend to be even more lax when it comes to pesticide control. Therefore, watch for domestic produce. Foods bought in season are generally domestic products.
- Beware of the "perfect" fruit or vegetable. Often the smaller, less pretty fruit or vegetable (as long as it is fresh and deep colored) is a product of fewer pesticides and chemicals used to improve the food's cosmetic appearance.
- Speak to the produce managers in the local supermarket. Ask them to list where the foods they sell are grown and which, if any, are organically grown without pesticides. Shop at chains such as California-based Raley's and Irving Ranch Farmers Market. These use independent testing laboratories to certify that their produce contains significantly reduced levels of pesticide residues.

Small-seeded fruits such as watermelon and pears may be juiced along with their skins, rinds, seeds, and cores. Large-seeded fruits such as papaya and peaches must part with their pits before juicing. Especially do not eat the pit of the apricot—it is poisonous to humans.

Most fruits and vegetables called for in the following recipes can be measured simply by sight. Sprouts and greens are a bit trickier. Measure sprouts, sunflower, and buckwheat greens by pressing gently into a measuring cup. Measure wheatgrass in "rounds," like spaghetti. A one-inch round of wheatgrass yields approximately one ounce of juice.

Once your fruits, vegetables, greens, and grasses have been cleaned and measured according to the guidelines here, cut them into pieces small enough to fit in the mouth of the appropriate juicer. Though it is necessary to cube carrots and similar root vegetables before juicing in a wheatgrass juicer, you may juice these vegetables uncut when you use a high-speed juicer.

Some recipes here call for juices to be strained before use. To strain pulp from juices, pour the blended mixture into a fine wire mesh strainer and tap the strainer on the top or sides while holding it over a glass or jar. Strained pulp may be discarded or, better yet, saved for compost.

When you have finished juicing, unplug and dismantle your juicer. Then, carefully clean it with a mild castile- or coconut-based soap and water. Thoroughly dry all parts before storing to prevent rust.

This chapter features five groups of juices: fresh fruit juices, fresh fruit smoothies, green drinks, wheatgrass drinks, and fresh vegetable juices. Each recipe yields approximately one 10-ounce glass of undiluted juice. To make a juice less strong or sweet-tasting, you may add spring water or sparkling water to it. All recipes in this chapter can be halved or doubled, as desired.

Though combinations of juices are highlighted in this chapter, juices squeezed from a single source are equally healthful and delicious. There is no reason why you can't enjoy a fruit, vegetable, sprout, wheatgrass, or green juice all by itself, unless otherwise specified in Chapters 4 and 5.

As a final note, don't forget to vary your use of fresh juices. Be creative: remember that juices can be used as bases for healthful and flavorful dressings, sauces, dips, and colorings of many varieties.

FRESH FRUIT JUICES

High in vitamins, minerals and other beneficial nutrients, fresh fruit juices are Nature's most delicious tonic. The recipes here combine tastes and textures in a host of fresh variations. Enjoy these fruity treats often—with meals or all by themselves, as energy boosters.

Apple Red-Eye

---

2 medium apples
4 handfuls cherries, pitted

Wash and slice apple. Combine with cherries. Juice and serve.

Grape-Apple

---

1 medium apple
1 small bunch grapes

Wash fruit. Remove grapes from stem. Slice apple. Combine with grapes. Juice and serve.

After the Fall
---

1 medium apple
1 medium pear, hard variety

Wash fruit. Combine. Juice and serve.

Apple Patch
---

2 medium apples
1 cup strawberries
1 teaspoon lemon juice

Wash fruit. Remove strawberry greens; discard. Combine with other ingredients. Juice and serve.

Mountain Punch
---

4 handfuls cherries, pitted
1 medium peach, pitted
1 medium pear, hard variety

Wash fruits. Combine. Juice and serve.

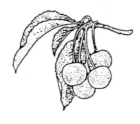

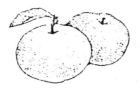

Cape Apple
---

2 medium apples
2 handfuls cranberries

Wash fruit. Combine. Juice and serve.

Mad Hatter
---

1 medium orange
½ grapefruit
2 handfuls cranberries

Wash fruits. Combine. Juice in high-speed juicer. Serve.

Grape Upper
---

1 small bunch grapes
½ papaya, peeled and pitted
1 teaspoon lemon juice

Wash fruits. Combine. Juice and serve.

Ape Juice

1 small bunch grapes
1 6-inch wedge peeled pineapple
1 teaspoon lime juice

Wash fruits. Combine. Juice and serve.

Citrus Surprise

½ grapefruit, pink or red
1 medium orange
1 cup strawberries

Wash fruit. Remove and discard strawberry greens. Combine fruits. Juice in high-speed juicer. Serve.

Mellow Mix

½ cantaloupe, meat only
½ cup honeydew melon, meat only
½ cup watermelon, meat and rind

Wash watermelon rind. Combine with other fruits. Juice and serve.

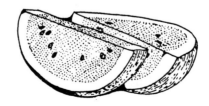

Prunapple

5-7 pitted prunes
1½ cups water
1 medium apple
½ pear, hard variety

Soak prunes overnight in one cup water. Combine prunes with soak water and remaining one-half cup water. Blend on high speed for two minutes. Strain prune pulp. Set juice aside. Wash other fruits. Combine, juice, and serve.

Strawberry Newton

1 medium apple
1-inch wedge peeled pineapple
1 cup strawberries

Wash fruits. Combine. Remove and discard strawberry greens. Juice and serve.

Orange Sun

½ papaya, peeled and pitted
1 medium peach, pitted
¼ grapefruit, red or pink

Wash fruits. Combine. Juice in high-speed juicer. Serve.

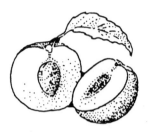

Summer Passion
---

1 medium peach, pitted
1 medium pear, hard variety
1 medium apple

Wash fruits. Juice and serve.

Tropical Cooler

2-inch wedge peeled pineapple
1 medium orange
1 tablespoon lemon juice

Wash fruits. Combine juice in high-speed juicer. Serve.

Daily Bread

2-inch wedge watermelon,
meat, rind, and seeds

Wash rind, juice, stir, and serve.

Winter Apple
---

3 medium apples
1 tablespoon ginger root, grated

Wash apple. Combine with grated ginger root. Juice. Serve in a warm glass.

FRESH FRUIT SMOOTHIES

Rich, frothy fruit smoothies are higher in vitamins and lower in calories than fast-food milkshakes. What's more, they taste great. The recipes that follow feature the freshest flavors this side of the orchard.

Orange Freeze
---

2 medium oranges
½ cup strawberries
½ banana

Wash strawberries, remove and discard greens. Peel banana. Freeze strawberries and banana. Juice oranges. Blend orange juice with frozen fruits on medium speed for one minute. Serve.

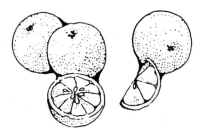

Tree Top

8 dried apricot halves
1 large apple
½ papaya, peeled and pitted

Soak apricots overnight in one cup water. Discard soak water
before juicing. Wash apple. Juice apple and papaya. Combine
apricots with apple/papaya juice. Blend for one minute on
medium speed. Serve.

Berry Nice

1 cup blueberries, frozen
2 medium pears, any variety

Wash fruit. Juice pears. Combine with berries. Blend at medium
speed for two minutes. Serve.

Morning Thunder

1 large peach, pitted
1 medium orange
½ banana

Wash peach. Combine with orange. Combine with banana.
Blend for one minute on medium speed. Serve for breakfast.

Pina Copaya

2-inch wedge peeled pineapple
½ papaya, peeled and pitted
⅔ cup fresh coconut meat, grated
½ cup water (optional)

Juice pineapple and papaya. Blend juice, coconut, and water on high speed for three minutes. Strain pulp; serve.

GREEN DRINKS

For the ultimate in healthfulness, there is no substitute for buckwheat and sunflower greens. However, when these are not available, sprouts may be substituted in the following green drink recipes.

Green drinks are best made in a wheatgrass juicer as many of the ingredients will oxidize (turn gray or brown) in high-speed juicers. If desired, strain green juice using a fine wire mesh strainer. Stir, and drink.

Basic Green Drink
---

1 cup buckwheat greens
1 cup sunflower greens
1 cup alfalfa sprouts
½ cup mung bean sprouts
1 medium carrot
1 stalk celery
½ medium cucumber
1 small scallion
2 tablespoons sauerkraut

Wash ingredients. Combine. Juice and serve.

A Plus

---

1 cup buckwheat greens
1 cup sunflower greens
1 cup alfalfa sprouts
½ cup cabbage sprouts
½ cup asparagus stems
3 kale leaves
1 medium carrot

Wash ingredients. Combine. Juice and serve.

Green Power

---

1 cup alfalfa sprouts
1 cup mung bean sprouts
¼ cup fenugreek sprouts
1 stalk celery
½ cucumber
3 beet greens
½ beet root
2 handfuls spinach
3 collard green leaves

Wash ingredients. Combine. Juice and serve.

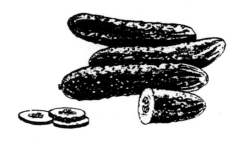

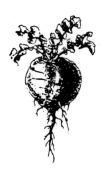

Wild Thing

---

1 cup sunflower greens
¼ cup radish sprouts
1 cup buckwheat greens
2 cups lamb's-quarters or purslane
1 stalk celery
½ small zucchini
½ green pepper
½ beet root

Wash ingredients. Combine. Juice and serve.

Blood Sugar Tonic

---

1 cup alfalfa sprouts
1 cup mung sprouts
1 cup lentil sprouts
2 kale leaves
1 cup Jerusalem artichokes
1 handful string beans
1 medium parsnip
½ cup fennel

Wash ingredients. Combine. Juice and serve.

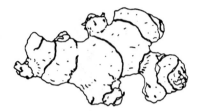

Hand Warmer
---

1 cup alfalfa sprouts
1 cup buckwheat greens
¼ cup radish sprouts
1 stalk celery
1 medium red pepper
1 medium parsnip
1 handful watercress
1 handful parsley
1 tablespoon fresh ginger root, grated

Wash ingredients. Combine. Juice. Serve in a warm glass.

Turn-Up Energy
---

1 cup sunflower greens
1 cup buckwheat greens
1 cup aduki bean sprouts
4 turnip green leaves
1 small yellow turnip
5 carrot tops
1 medium carrot
½ cup fennel

Wash ingredients. Combine. Juice and serve.

WHEATGRASS DRINKS

In the recipes that follow, there is no substitute for wheatgrass. Each should be prepared in a wheatgrass juicer, unless specified otherwise. Because it spoils quickly, wheatgrass in the following drink recipes should be juiced after all other ingredients to ensure you are getting the freshest drink possible. Measure wheatgrass in "rounds," like spaghetti. A one-inch round of wheatgrass will yield about one ounce of juice.

Green Machine

---

2 handfuls parsley
2- to 3-inch round wheatgrass
2 ounces water

Wash greens. Juice and combine with water. Serve in shot glasses.

Wheatgrasshopper

3-inch wedge peeled pineapple
1 sprig mint
2- to 3-inch round wheatgrass

Wash wheatgrass. Juice pineapple and mint in high-speed juicer. Juice wheatgrass in wheatgrass juice. Combine and serve.

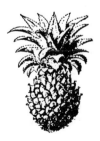

Salty Grass
---

5 stalks celery
2- to 3-inch round wheatgrass

Wash ingredients. Combine. Juice and serve.

Veggie Grass
---

2 medium carrots
3 stalks celery
1 handful parsley
1 handful watercress
½ beet root
½ cup fennel
2- to 3-inch round wheatgrass

Wash ingredients. Combine. Juice and serve.

FRESH VEGETABLE DRINKS

All fresh vegetable recipes that follow can be made in a high-speed juicer. Feel free to adjust or add to the recipes according to your tastes. Green-, sprout-, or wheatgrass juices are but a few possible additions. As with fruits, the freshest vegetables will yield the most healthful juices. Fresh vegetable juices will keep two to three days in the refrigerator.

Spring 8

½ cup asparagus
4 medium carrots
1 radish
2 handfuls spinach
4 collard leaves
3 stalks celery
1 cup watercress
1 scallion

Wash ingredients. Combine. Juice and serve.

Fall 8
---

3 medium parsnips
1 cup Jerusalem artichokes
5 leaves kale
1 cup cabbage
5 leaves lettuce
3 stalks celery
3 handfuls spinach
1 scallion

Wash ingredients. Combine. Juice and serve.

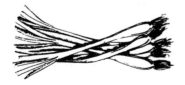

Sweet Heart

5 medium carrots
1 small apple
½ medium beet

Wash ingredients. Combine. Juice and serve.

Cabbage Patch

¼ head cabbage
2 stalks celery
1 cup fennel

Wash ingredients. Combine. Juice and serve.

Hair Food

6 lettuce leaves
3 handfuls spinach
3 medium carrots
1 cup cabbage
4 kale leaves
½ cup fennel

Wash ingredients. Combine. Juice and serve.

Pepperoni

1 large green pepper, stem removed
1 large red pepper, stem removed
3 celery stalks
⅓ medium cucumber
5 lettuce leaves

Wash ingredients. Combine. Juice and serve.

Skin Trip

2 medium carrots
½ medium cucumber
½ medium green pepper
1 handful watercress
2 handfuls spinach
3 kale leaves

Wash ingredients. Combine. Juice and serve.

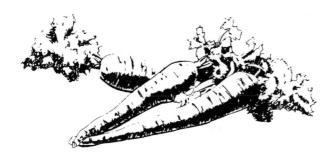

Eight-Vegetable Drink

½ medium tomato
¼ medium cucumber
1 medium carrot
1 stalk celery
1 handful spinach
½ medium red pepper
½ cup cabbage
1 scallion

Wash ingredients. Combine. Juice and serve.

Mock Tomato

2 medium carrots
½ medium beet root
2 stalks celery
1 cup mung sprouts

Wash ingredients. Combine. Juice and serve.

Nice 'N Sweet

2 medium carrots
½ medium apple
¼ medium beet
1 celery stalk
½ medium pear, hard variety
¼ cup fennel

Wash ingredients. Combine. Juice and serve.

Red Hot

3 radishes
¼ cup radish sprouts
½ medium beet
½ medium sweet red pepper
½ medium cucumber

Wash ingredients. Combine. Juice and serve.

Cressida

3 handfuls watercress
3 stalks celery
1 medium parsnip
½ medium green pepper,
    stem removed
1 cup fennel

Wash ingredients. Combine. Juice and serve.

Let-Us Drink

6 lettuce leaves
2 celery stalks
1 large apple

Wash ingredients. Combine. Juice and serve.

Popeye's Pride

5 handfuls spinach
1 medium cucumber
2 medium carrots

Wash ingredients. Combine. Juice and serve.

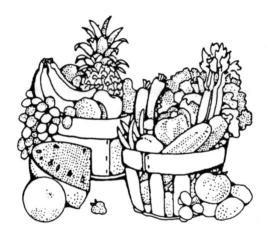

8
Choosing Bottled Juices

Although this book recommends the use of juices made fresh at home, bottled juices—not canned or in cartons—can be a healthful alternative to artificial and sugar-sweetened drinks such as coffee, soft drinks, wine, and beer. This chapter lists the manufacturers that provide both the purest and most nutritious bottled juices, and discusses why their juices are superior.

WHAT IS NATURAL JUICE?

Today in the United States the term "natural" can be applied to almost any packaged juice. But savvy shoppers who read labels will note that there are definite degrees of "naturalness."

To be labeled "natural," the United States Food and Drug Administration (FDA) requires that a juice contain no artificial colors, sweeteners, or preservatives. But the FDA's definition of "artificial" excludes some major nutritional villains. According to the FDA, white sugar is "natural." So are juice concentrates, juices extracted using chemical methods, and filtered juices. Understandably, many consumers are questioning the best way to choose a nutritious juice, with such a wide selection of so-called "natural" juices on the market.

The most healthful natural juices are relatively unfiltered. They have a cloudy appearance. The sediment that forms on the bottom of the bottle is made up of tiny particles of fruit. This indicates to the consumer that more whole fruit has been used to make the juice. Thicker, cloudier juices provide greater nutrition than thinner, clearer juices. What's more, they taste better.

Although clear, filtered juices, and those made exclusively from concentrates may be labeled "100-percent-natural," they are best avoided. This is because with them you don't always know what you are getting. For example, you will recall from the Introduction that Beech-Nut Nutrition Corp. was recently indicted for selling sugar-water labeled 100-percent apple juice. That section also detailed how juice manufacturers of national brands reconstitute imported fruit juice concentrates with tap water from industrial park sites. Still other juice companies use chemical means to extract juice from fruit and vegetables. Or they spoil a good product by packaging their juices in cans or cartons.

Canned juices are not recommended. When acids from the juice leech metal from the can, the juice can spoil. Similarly, juices that are packed in cartons are in direct contact with the wax and chemicals used to make the paper container they are packed in. Juices packed in cartons that are shrink-wrapped are exposed to high heat used in the shrink-wrap process. For these reasons, juice products that come in cans and cartons are not recommended. Sterilized, vacuum-sealed glass bottles remain the superior choice as juice containers.

THE BEST MASS PRODUCERS OF BOTTLED JUICES

Because they adhere to strict standards of cleanliness and quality control, bottled juices manufactured by the following reputable companies are recommended. These companies do their best to provide high-quality products made from high-quality produce, using high-quality methods.

Each of these companies offers juices with minimal filtration, leaving the juices with a rich, cloudy appearance. The cloudiness and sediment at the bottom of their juices is caused by an abundance of small pieces of fruit that get through the filters. This sediment makes the juice more nutritious and flavorful. All of the juice companies listed also go out of their way to obtain the freshest, least sprayed, and most flavorful fruits to juice. For each listed here, the emphasis is not on appearance and shelf life but, rather, on quality, freshness, and flavor.

After the Fall

A New York-based company that distributes to many supermarkets and natural foods stores, mostly east of the Mississippi River. Their line of more than fifteen juices is dominated by apple blends. *After the Fall*'s apple-strawberry and pear juices are excellent. You'll want to try their natural lemonade, as well.

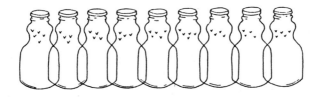

Apple and Eve

Another New York-based company, Apple and Eve pledges their products contain only 100-percent-pure juice. Their apple juice is made from apples grown in upstate New York. Like *After the Fall*, they offer tasty apple juice blends. Especially good are their Cape Cod varieties of cranberry and apple juices. *Apple and Eve* juice has a rich flavor and a characteristically cloudy appearance. It is available in most supermarkets in the eastern United States.

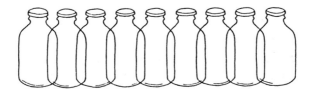

Eden

Based in Michigan, *Eden* specializes in fruit juices made from fruits grown in the Midwest. Cherry, apple, prune, Concord grape, and several tasty apple blends comprise their juice line. *Eden* juice products can be purchased in most natural foods stores and some supermarkets in the Midwest and on the East Coast.

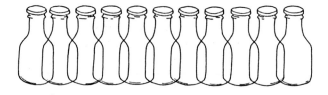

Heinke's

One of the finest and perhaps oldest of the natural juice companies, *Heinke's* is located in California. A dozen pure fruit juices made without concentrates and nearly twenty fruit juice blends comprise their juice line. The company grows its own grapes to make its delicious Concord grape juice. *Heinke's* juices are sold in some supermarkets and many natural foods stores throughout the U.S.

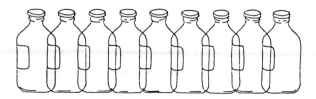

Lakewood

The sunny taste of the South characterizes these exotic fruit juice blends. A Florida-based juice maker, *Lakewood* specializes in tropical blends, while producing more than three dozen varieties. They offer no less than seven papaya blends. Other exotic choices are juices of guavas, mangos, and coconuts. *Lakewood* also produces apple and berry blends that are typical of the Northern juice producers. *Lakewood* juices can be found in natural foods stores nationwide.

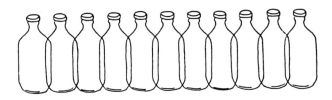

R. W. Knudsen

Another California juice maker, *Knudsen* offers a greater variety of juices than any other company—nearly sixty in all. Their tasty line includes seven pure grape juice varieties, several other single-fruit varieties, dozens of juice blends including several exotic concoctions, and herb coolers made from juices and herb teas. You can purchase *Knudsen* juices in supermarkets and natural foods stores nationwide.

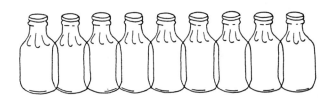

Walnut Acres

Pennsylvania-based *Walnut Acres* is an organic and whole foods company that offers a variety of quality juices. Extracted from. organically grown grapes, apples, and cranberries, *Walnut Acres* juices have a richness and flavor that is worthy of praise. Several other varieties are available, as well. Though *Walnut Acres* juice has a limited distribution nationwide, don't assume they're not sold in your area. Look for them in more discriminating natural foods stores near you.

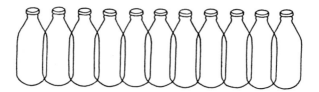

Winter Hill

This East Coast producer is the natural juice subsidiary of Lincoln Foods Company which also produces the *Lincoln* juice line. Unlike the *Lincoln* juice line, however, *Winter Hill* juices are minimally filtered and full-flavored. More than twenty varieties of pure fruit juice and juice blends carry the *Winter Hill* label. Their apple blends are especially tasty. *Winter Hill* juices can be found in supermarkets and natural foods stores nationwide.

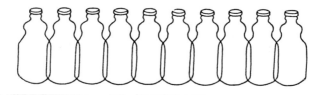

Conclusion

A Toast to
Your Good Health

Combined with a balanced diet, regular exercise, and a positive attitude, the juices of sprouts, greens, wheatgrass, fresh vegetables, and fresh fruits can play an important role in attaining and maintaining good health. Quite simply, these foods have the power to protect us from illness by strengthening our immune systems. They stimulate our overall metabolism, keep us clean and balanced inside, and mobilize our body's defenses against a myriad of modern-day environmental stresses that have been shown to cause degenerative disease.

In this Modern Age, biological mechanisms like the human body cannot thrive, or even survive, on synthetic processed foods and chemicals, though these constitute more than half of the present diet in the Western World. Observing the pale complexions, lethargic movement, and ill health of those who eat this way, one can only guess the long-term effect this type of diet will have on the world's population—if left unchecked. It has been said that the disappearance of live foods from the modern diet lowers the quality of life for all Earth's inhabitants to a greater or lesser extent. But we do have choices. By switching to a live foods diet that includes plenty of fresh fruit and vegetable juices, we can each do our part not only to increase our own healthfulness, but to add momentum to a positive trend, as well.

At present, there is a well-grounded movement towards "natural" foods and body care products in the United States. And though this shift in consciousness has been slow moving, it is definitely heading in the right direction. Good examples all, many prominent nutritionists, political leaders, entertainers, and physicians are leading the way by living a more natural lifestyle.

These health-conscious people know that no amount of surgery, pills, therapy, or money can keep us well. Only a desire and willingness to understand and put in practice Nature's laws can do so. This means that we must eat plenty of live, raw foods such as fruits, vegetables, sprouts, and greens, and their juices, with all of their vital nutrients intact.

Growing and juicing our own fruits, vegetables, sprouts, and greens is not only a healthful alternative to drinking soft drinks, coffee, teas, and alcoholic beverages. It's a fun way for the whole family to focus on health. Far from a frivolous impracticality, squeezing fresh juices at home can easily become a focal point of your family's health program. Ounce for ounce, fresh fruit and vegetable juices are both more nutritious and less expensive than other beverages. A juicer that's right for your family's needs will pay for itself many times over in doctors' bills you'll save by making a variety of fresh-squeezed juices part of your daily diet.

Now that you've learned about the important role fresh juices play in cleansing, building, and restoring your body, what are you waiting for? Better health can be just a sip away. Bottoms up!

Appendix A

JUICE NUTRIENT
TROUBLESHOOTING CHART

Vitamin	Bodily Action
Bioflavonoids	Help to increase strength of capillaries.
Choline	Important in nerve transmission, metabolism of fats. Helps regulate liver and gall bladder.
Folic acid (folacin)	Important in red blood cell formation. Aids metabolism of protein necessary for growth and division of body cells.
Inositol	Necessary for formation of the phospholipid lecithin which is connected with the metabolism of fats including cholesterol. Vital for hair growth.
Niacin (nicotinic acid, niacinimide)	Maintains health of skin, tongue, and digestive system. Essential for utilization of carbohydrate, fat, and protein.
PABA (Para aminobenzoic acid)	Aids bacteria in production of folic acid. Acts as a co-enzyme in the breakdown and utilization of proteins. Aids in formation of red blood cells. Acts as a sunscreen.
Pantothenic acid	Aids in formation of some fats, participates in the release of energy from carbohydrates, fats, and protein. Improves body's resistance to stress.

Deficiency Symptoms	Source
Tendency to bleed and bruise easily.	Citrus fruits, black currants.
Fatty liver, bleeding kidneys, high blood pressure.	Green vegetables.
Poor growth, anemia, vitamin B_{12} deficiency.	Dark green leafy vegetables. Asparagus, broccoli, sprouts, root vegetables, Brussels sprouts.
Constipation, eczema, hair loss, elevated cholesterol.	Citrus fruits, green vegetables.
Dermatitis, nervous disorders.	Dates, broccoli, herbs.
Fatigue, irritability, depression, nervousness, constipation, headache, digestive disorders, grey hair.	Asparagus, broccoli, sprouts, root vegetables, Brussels sprouts, dark green leafy vegetables.
Vomiting, restlessness, stomach stress, increased susceptibility to infection.	Broccoli, cabbage, cauliflower.

JUICE NUTRIENT
TROUBLESHOOTING CHART (CONTINUED)

Vitamin	Bodily Action
Vitamin A	Necessary for growth and repair of body tissue, eyes, and eyesight. Fights bacteria and infection, maintains healthy epithelial tissue, aids bone and teeth formation.
Vitamin B Complex	Necessary for carbohydrate, fat, and protein metabolism. Helps functioning of the nervous system, muscle tone in gastro-intestinal tract.
Vitamin B-1	Maintains health of skin, hair, eyes, mouth, and liver. Necessary for carbohydrate metabolism. Maintains healthy nervous system. Stimulates growth and muscle tone.
Vitamin B-2	Necessary for carbohydrate, fat, and protein metabolism. Aids in formation of antibodies and red blood cells. Maintains respiration.
Vitamin B-6 (pyridoxine)	Necessary for carbohydrate, fat, and protein metabolism. Aids in formation of antibodies. Maintains balance of sodium and phosphorus.
Vitamin C	Maintains collagen, helps heal wounds, scar tissue, and fractures. Gives strength to blood vessels. Provides resistance to stress.

Deficiency Symptoms	Source
Night blindness, rough, dry skin, fatigue, loss of smell and appetite.	Yellow fruits and vegetables.
Dry, rough, cracked skin; acne; dull, dry or grey hair; poor appetite; stomach disorders.	Sprouts, greens, citrus fruits.
Gastrointestinal problems, fatigue, loss of appetite, nerve disorders, heart disorders.	Asparagus, beans, pineapple, herbs.
Eye problems, cracks and sores in mouth, dermatitis, retarded growth, digestive disturbances.	Baby green vegetables, broccoli, asparagus, herbs.
Anemia, mouth disorders, nervousness, muscular weakness, dermatitis, edema, allergies.	Green leafy vegetables.
Bleeding gums, swollen or painful joints, slow healing of wounds and fractures, bruising, nosebleeds, impaired digestion.	Citrus fruits, alfalfa sprouts, cantaloupe, strawberries, broccoli, green peppers, tomatoes.

JUICE NUTRIENT
TROUBLESHOOTING CHART (CONTINUED)

Vitamin	Bodily Action
Vitamin E	Protects fat-soluble vitamins and red blood cells. Essential in cellular respiration. Inhibits coagulation of blood.
Vitamin K	Necessary for blood coagulation.

Mineral	Bodily Action
Calcium	Essential for development and maintenance of strong bones and teeth. Assists normal blood clotting, muscle action, nerve function, and heart function.
Cobalt	Functions as part of vitamin B-12. Maintains red blood cells. Activates a number of enzymes in the body.
Copper	Aids in formation of red blood cells. Forms part of many enzymes. Works with vitamin C to form the protein elastin.
Iodine	Essential part of the hormone thyroxine. Necessary for prevention of goiter. Regulates energy and metabolism. Promotes growth.

Deficiency Symptoms	Source
Rupture of red blood cells, muscular wasting, abnormal fat deposits in muscles.	Leeks, cabbage, Brussels sprouts, herbs, sprouts, green leafy vegetables.
Increased tendency to hemorrhage and miscarriage.	Cauliflower, green leafy vegetables.

Deficiency Symptoms	Source
Softening of bones, back and leg pains, brittle bones.	Green leafy vegetables, especially kale.
Pernicious anemia, slow rate of growth.	Green vegetables, ripe fruits.
General weakness, impaired respiration, skin sores.	Green vegetables.
Weakness, pale skin, constipation, anemia.	Pineapple, green leafy vegetables.

JUICE NUTRIENT
TROUBLESHOOTING CHART (CONTINUED)

Mineral	Bodily Action
Iron	Necessary for hemoglobin and myoglobin formation. Helps protein metabolism. Promotes growth.
Magnesium	Acts as a catalyst in the utilization of carbohydrates, fat, protein, calcium, phosphorus, and potassium.
Manganese	Activates enzymes. Necessary for normal skeletal development. Maintains sex hormone production.

Deficiency Symptoms	Source
Weakness, paleness of skin, constipation, anemia.	Asparagus, bing cherries, apricots, black raspberries, prunes.
Nervousness, muscular excitability, tremors.	Dark green vegetables.
Paralysis, convulsions, dizziness, ataxia, blindness and deafness in infants.	Apples, apricots, pineapple, green leafy vegetables.

Appendix B

NUTRIENT COMPOSITION FOR SELECTED FRUITS AND VEGETABLES
(PER 3½ OUNCE PORTION)

	PROTEIN	FAT	CARBOHYDRATE	CALCIUM	PHOSPHORUS
	Gm	Gm	Gm	Mg	Mg
Apples	.2	.6	14.5	7	10
Apricots	1.0	.2	12.8	17	23
Artichokes	2.0	.2	10.6	51	88
Asparagus	2.5	.2	5.0	22	62
Avocados	2.1	16.4	6.3	10	42
Bananas	1.1	.2	22.2	8	26
Beans (White)	22.3	1.6	61.3	144	425
Beans (Pinto)	22.9	1.2	63.7	135	457
Beans (Lima)	8.4	.5	22.1	52	142
Beans (Mung)	24.2	1.3	60.3	118	340
Beans (Snap)	1.9	.2	7.1	56	44
Beans (Mung Sprouts)	3.8	.2	6.6	19	64
Beet (Red)	1.6	.1	9.9	16	33
Beet (Greens)	2.2	.3	4.6	119	40
Blackberries	1.2	.9	12.9	32	19
Blueberries	.7	.5	15.3	15	13
Breadfruit	1.7	.3	26.2	33	32

IRON	SODIUM	POTASSIUM	VITAMIN A	THIAMINE B-1	RIBOFLAVIN B-2	NIACIN	ASCORBIC ACID
Mg	Mg	Mg	Mg	IU	Mg	Mg	Mg
.3	1	110	90	.03	.02	.1	4
.5	1	281	2700	.03	.04	.6	10
1.3	43	430	160	.08	.05	1.0	12
1.0	2	278	900	.18	.20	1.5	33
.6	4	604	290	.11	.20	1.6	14
.7	1	370	190	.05	.06	.7	10
7.8	19	1196	0	.65	.22	2.4	—
6.4	10	984	—	.84	.21	2.2	—
2.8	2	650	290	.24	.12	1.4	29
7.7	6	1028	80	.38	.21	2.6	—
.8	7	243	600	.08	.11	.5	19
1.3	5	223	20	.13	.13	.8	19
.7	60	335	20	.03	.05	.4	10
3.3	130	570	6100	.10	.22	.4	30
.9	1	170	200	.03	.04	.4	21
1.0	1	81	100	.03	.06	.5	14
1.2	15	439	40	.11	.03	.9	29

NUTRIENT COMPOSITION FOR SELECTED FRUITS AND VEGETABLES
(PER 3½ OUNCE PORTION, CONTINUED)

	PROTEIN Gm	FAT Gm	CARBOHYDRATE Gm	CALCIUM Mg	PHOSPHORUS Mg
Cabbage	1.3	.2	5.4	49	29
Carrots	1.1	.2	9.7	37	36
Cauliflower	2.7	.2	5.2	25	56
Celery	.9	.1	3.9	39	28
Chard (Swiss)	2.4	.3	4.6	88	39
Cherries (Sweet)	1.3	.3	17.4	22	19
Chives	1.8	.3	5.8	69	44
Collards	4.8	.8	7.5	250	82
Corn (Field)	8.9	3.9	72.2	22	268
Corn (Sweet)	3.5	1	22.1	3	111
Crabapples	.4	.3	17.8	6	13
Eggplant	1.2	.2	5.6	12	26
Elderberries	2.6	.5	16.4	38	28
Endive	1.7	.1	4.1	81	54
Figs	1.2	.3	20.3	35	22
Garlic	6.2	.2	30.8	29	202
Gooseberries	.8	.2	9.7	18	15

IRON	SODIUM	POTASSIUM	VITAMIN A	THIAMINE B-1	RIBOFLAVIN B-2	NIACIN	ASCORBIC ACID
Mg	Mg	Mg	Mg	IU	Mg	Mg	Mg
.4	20	233	130	.05	.05	.3	47
.7	47	341	11000	.06	.05	.6	8
1.1	13	295	60	.11	.10	.7	78
.3	126	341	240	.03	.03	3	9
3.2	147	550	6500	.06	.17	.5	32
.4	2	191	110	.05	.06	.4	10
1.7	—	250	5800	.08	.13	.5	56
1.5	—	450	9300	.16	.31	1.7	152
2.1	1	284	490	.37	.12	2.2	0
.7	Trace	280	400	.15	.12	1.7	12
.3	1	110	40	.03	.02	.1	8
.7	2	214	10	.05	.05	.6	5
1.6	—	300	600	.07	.06	.5	36
1.7	14	294	3300	.07	.14	.5	10
.6	2	194	80	.06	.05	.4	2
1.5	19	529	Trace	.25	.08	.5	15
.5	1	155	290	—	—	—	33

NUTRIENT COMPOSITION FOR SELECTED FRUITS AND VEGETABLES
(PER 3½ OUNCE PORTION, CONTINUED)

	PROTEIN	FAT	CARBOHYDRATE	CALCIUM	PHOSPHORUS
	Gm	Gm	Gm	Mg	Mg
Grapefruit	.5	.1	10.6	16	16
Grapes	1.3	.1	15.7	16	12
Guavas	.8	.6	15.0	23	42
Kale	6.0	8	9	249	93
Kumquats	.9	.1	17.1	63	23
Leeks	2.2	.3	11.2	52	50
Lemons	1.1	.3	8.2	26	16
Lentils	24.7	1.1	60.1	79	377
Lettuce	1.2	.2	2.5	35	26
Mushrooms	2.7	.3	4.4	6	116
Muskmelons	.7	.1	7.5	14	16
Mustard greens	3.0	.5	5.6	183	50
Nectarines	.6	Trace	17.1	4	24
Okra	2.4	.3	7.6	92	51
Onions (Dry)	1.5	.1	8.7	27	36
Onions (Green)	1.5	.2	8.2	51	39
Oranges	1.0	.2	12.2	41	20

IRON	SODIUM	POTASSIUM	VITAMIN A	THIAMINE B-1	RIBOFLAVIN B-2	NIACIN	ASCORBIC ACID
Mg	Mg	Mg	Mg	IU	Mg	Mg	Mg
.4	1	135	80	.04	.02	.2	38
.4	3	158	100	.05	.03	.3	4
.9	4	289	280	.05	.05	1.2	242
2.7	75	378	10000	.16	.26	2.1	186
.4	7	236	600	.08	.10	—	36
1.1	5	347	40	.11	.06	.5	17
.6	2	138	20	.04	.02	.1	53
6.8	30	790	60	.37	.22	2	—
2.0	9	264	970	.06	.06	.3	8
.8	15	414	Trace	.10	.46	4.2	3
.4	12	251	3400	.04	.03	.6	33
3.0	32	377	7000	.11	.22	.8	97
.5	6	294	1650	—	—	—	13
.6	3	249	520	.17	.21	1.0	31
.5	10	157	40	.03	.04	.2	10
1.0	5	231	2000	.05	.05	.4	32
.4	1	200	200.	.10	.04	.4	50

NUTRIENT COMPOSITION FOR SELECTED FRUITS AND VEGETABLES
(PER 3½ OUNCE PORTION, CONTINUED)

	PROTEIN Gm	FAT Gm	CARBOHYDRATE Gm	CALCIUM Mg	PHOSPHORUS Mg
Papayas	.6	.1	10.0	20	16
Parsley	3.6	.6	8.5	203	63
Parsnips	1.7	.5	17.5	50	77
Peaches	.6	.1	9.7	9	19
Pears	.7	.4	15.3	8	11
Peas (Edible pod)	3.4	.2	12.0	62	90
Peas (Green)	6.3	.4	14.4	26	116
Peppers (Hot red)	3.7	2.3	18.1	29	78
Peppers (Sweet green)	1.2	.2	4.8	9	22
Persimmons	.7	.4	19.7	6	26
Pineapple	.4	.2	13.7	17	8
Plums	.5	Trace	17.8	18	17
Pomegranate	.5	.3	16.4	3	8
Potatoes	2.1	.1	17.1	7	53
Rhubarb	.6	.1	3.7	96	18
Spinach	3.2	.3	4.3	93	51
Squash	1.1	.1	4.2	28	29

IRON	SODIUM	POTASSIUM	VITAMIN A	THIAMINE B-1	RIBOFLAVIN B-2	NIACIN	ASCORBIC ACID
Mg	Mg	Mg	Mg	IU	Mg	Mg	Mg
.3	3	234	1750	.04	.04	.3	56
6.2	45	727	8500	.12	.26	1.2	172
.7	12	541	30	.08	.09	.2	16
.5	1	202	1330	.02	.05	1.0	7
.3	2	130	20	.02	.04	.1	4
.7	—	170	680	.28	.12	—	21
1.9	2	316	640	.35	.14	2.9	27
1.2	—	—	21600	.22	.36	4.4	369
.7	13	213	420	.08	.08	.5	128
.3	6	174	2700	.03	.02	.1	11
.5	1	146	70	.09	.03	.2	17
.5	2	299	300	.08	.03	.5	—
.3	3	259	Trace	.03	.03	.3	4
.6	3	407	Trace	.10	.04	1.5	20
.8	2	251	100	.03	.07	.3	9
3.1	71	470	8100	.10	.20	.6	51
.4	1	202	410	.05	.09	1.0	22

NUTRIENT COMPOSITION FOR SELECTED FRUITS AND VEGETABLES
(PER 3½ OUNCE PORTION, CONTINUED)

	PROTEIN Gm	FAT Gm	CARBOHYDRATE Gm	CALCIUM Mg	PHOSPHORUS Mg
Strawberries	.7	.5	8.4	21	21
Sweet Potatoes	1.7	.4	26.3	32	47
Tangerines	.8	.2	11.6	40	18
Tomatoes	1.1	.2	4.7	13	27
Turnips	1.0	.2	6.6	39	30
Turnip (Greens)	3.0	.3	5.0	246	58
Watercress	2.2	.3	3.0	151	54
Watermelon	.5	.2	6.4	7	10

Source: *Composition of Foods Handbook #8.* U.S. Department of Agriculture.

IRON Mg	SODIUM Mg	POTASSIUM Mg	VITAMIN A Mg	THIAMINE B-1 IU	RIBOFLAVIN B-2 Mg	NIACIN Mg	ASCORBIC ACID Mg
1.0	1	164	60	.03	.07	.6	59
.7	10	243	8800	.10	.06	.6	21
.4	2	126	420	.06	.02	.1	31
.5	3	244	900	.06	.04	.7	23
.5	49	268	Trace	.04	.07	.6	36
1.8	—	—	7600	.21	.39	.8	139
1.7	52	282	4900	.08	.16	.9	79
.5	1	100	590	.03	.03	.2	7

Index

Alfalfa sprout
juice, 38–39. *See also* Conditions
treated with fresh vegetable
juices; Minerals, sources of;
Vitamins, sources of.
juice recipes, 117, 118, 119, 120
Amino acids, 11–12
Apple
juice, 80–82. *See also* Conditions
treated with fresh fruit juices.
juice recipes, 109, 110, 111, 113,
114, 115, 116, 124, 126, 127
nutrient composition of, 148–149.
See also Minerals, sources of;
Vitamins, sources of.
Apricot
frozen fruit juice recipe, 117
nutrient composition of, 148–149.
See also Minerals, sources of.
Artichoke
juice, 39–40. *See also* Conditions
treated with fresh vegetable
juices.
juice recipes, 119, 123
nutrient composition of, 148–149.
See also Minerals, sources of;
Vitamins, sources of.
Asparagus
juice, 40–41. *See also* Conditions
treated with fresh vegetable
juices.
juice recipes, 118, 123
nutrient composition of, 148–149.
See also Minerals, sources of;
Vitamins, sources of.

Banana
frozen fruit juice recipe, 116
nutrient composition of,
148–149.
Bean sprout
juice, 41–42. *See also* Conditions
treated with fresh vegetable
juices.
juice recipes, 117, 118, 119,
120, 126
nutrient composition of, 148–149.
See also Minerals, sources of;
Vitamins, sources of.
Beet and beet green
juice, 42–43. *See also* Conditions
treated with fresh vegetable
juices.
juice recipes, 118, 119, 122, 124,
126, 127
nutrient composition of, 148–149.
See also Minerals, sources of;
Vitamins, sources of.
Blender, function of, 22–23
Blueberry
frozen fruit juice recipe, 117
nutrient composition of, 148–149
Buckwheat and buckwheat green
juice, 43–44. *See also* Conditions
treated with fresh vegetable
juices; Minerals, sources of;
Vitamins, sources of.
juice recipes, 117, 118, 119, 120
nutrient composition of, 148–149.
See also Minerals, sources of;
Vitamins, sources of.